Clinical Immunobiology

VOLUME 4

Clinical Immunobiology

Edited by

VOLUME 4

FRITZ H. BACH, M.D.
IMMUNOBIOLOGY RESEARCH CENTER
DEPARTMENTS OF MEDICAL GENETICS
AND SURGERY
UNIVERSITY OF WISCONSIN
MADISON, WISCONSIN

ROBERT A. GOOD, Ph.D., M.D.
MEMORIAL SLOAN–KETTERING
CANCER CENTER
NEW YORK, NEW YORK

ACADEMIC PRESS
A Subsidiary of Harcourt Brace Jovanovich, Publishers
New York   London   Toronto   Sydney   San Francisco   1980

COPYRIGHT © 1980, BY ACADEMIC PRESS, INC.
ALL RIGHTS RESERVED.
NO PART OF THIS PUBLICATION MAY BE REPRODUCED OR
TRANSMITTED IN ANY FORM OR BY ANY MEANS, ELECTRONIC
OR MECHANICAL, INCLUDING PHOTOCOPY, RECORDING, OR ANY
INFORMATION STORAGE AND RETRIEVAL SYSTEM, WITHOUT
PERMISSION IN WRITING FROM THE PUBLISHER.

ACADEMIC PRESS, INC.
111 Fifth Avenue, New York, New York 10003

United Kingdom Edition published by
ACADEMIC PRESS, INC. (LONDON) LTD.
24/28 Oval Road, London NW1 7DX

LIBRARY OF CONGRESS CATALOG CARD NUMBER: 72-77356

ISBN 0-12-070004-2

PRINTED IN THE UNITED STATES OF AMERICA

80 81 82 83   9 8 7 6 5 4 3 2 1

Contents

List of Contributors	xi
Preface	xv
Contents of Previous Volumes	xix

General Orientation of Human Lymphocyte Subpopulations

Sudhir Gupta, Robert J. Winchester, and Robert A. Good

I. Introduction	2
II. Cytoplasmic Immunoglobulin	5
III. Membrane Immunoglobulin	6
IV. Ia System	9
V. Epstein–Barr Virus (EBV) Receptor	12
VI. Complement Receptors	13
VII. Receptors for Fc Region of Immunoglobulins	14
VIII. Enzymatic Markers	17
IX. Receptors for Peanut Agglutinin	18
X. Erythrocyte Receptors	19
XI. Surface Antigens of Lymphocyte Subpopulations Defined by Monoclonal Antibodies	21
XII. Relationship between Tγ Cells and Monocytes	26
XIII. Distinction of Lymphocytes from Monocytes	28
XIV. The Third-Cell Population or Unclassified Lymphoid Cells	29
XV. Summary	30
References	30

Lymphocyte Membrane Complement Receptors
Gordon D. Ross

I. Introduction	33
II. Methods for Detection of C Receptors	37
III. Expression of C Receptors and Other Surface Markers on Normal and Leukemic Human Lymphocytes	40
IV. Interpetation and Significance	42
References	45

Regulatory Human T-Cell Subpopulations Defined by Receptors for IgG or IgM
Lorenzo Moretta and Max D. Cooper

I. Introduction	47
II. Enumeration and Isolation of T_M and T_G Cells	48
III. Morphology of T_M and T_G Cells	49
IV. Tissue Distribution of T_M and T_G Cells	50
V. Functional Analysis of T_M and T_G Cells	50
VI. Clinical Relevance of T_M and T_G Subpopulations	52
Selected Reading	53
Addendum	53

Mitogens
John D. Stobo

I. Introduction	55
II. Fundamentals of Lectin-Induced Mitogenesis	57
III. Procedure for Determining *in Vitro* Lectin-Induced Activation of Lymphocytes	62
IV. Clinical Usefulness of Lectins	65
General Reading References	72

Natural Killer Cells and Cells Mediating Antibody-Dependent Cytotoxicity against Tumors
Ronald B. Herberman

I. Introduction	73
II. Methods	74
III. Characteristics of NK Cells and Their Relationship to K Cells	77

IV. Specificity of Natural Cytotoxicity	79
V. Factors Affecting Levels of NK and K Cell Activities	82
VI. Possible Clinical Significance of These Effector Cells	84
References	86

Regulation of the Immune System by Lymphocyte Sets: Analysis in Animal Models

H. Cantor

I. General Considerations	89
II. Analysis in the Mouse	91
III. Conclusions	95
Selected References	97

The Serology of HLA-A, -B, and -C

F. Kissmeyer-Nielsen

I. Introduction	99
II. Experimental Methods and Findings	100
III. Conclusions	109
References	111

The Serology of HLA-DR

J. J. van Rood and A. van Leeuwen

I. Introduction	113
II. Technical Considerations	114
III. Results	118
IV. Discussion	120
References	121

Cellular Immunogenetics—Definition of HLA-D Region Encoded Antigens by T Lymphocyte Reactivities

Fritz H. Bach and Paul M. Sondel

I. Introduction	124
II. Mixed Leukocyte Culture Homozygous Typing Cells	127
III. Primed LD-Typing (PLT)	132
IV. General Discussion	141
References	142

Cell-Mediated Lympholysis

Dolores J. Schendel

I. Introduction	143
II. Terminology	145
III. Technique	146
IV. Specificity of Cell-Mediated Lympholysis	147
V. Genetic Control of CML	148
VI. Cell-Mediated Lympholysis Typing	151
VII. Preliminary Information from CML Typing Experiments	157
VIII. Future Prospects	158
Suggested Reading List	160

HLA and Graft Survival

J. J. van Rood and G. G. Persijn

I. Introduction	161
II. Methodology	164
III. Results	166
IV. Discussion	170
References	171

HLA and Disease

A. Svejgaard and L. P. Ryder

I. Introduction	173
II. Methods	174
III. Relationships between HLA and Diseases	175
IV. Disease Heterogeneity	176
V. Inheritance of Disease Susceptibility and Resistance	177
VI. Mechanisms that Can Explain the Associations	179
VII. Diagnostic and Prognostic Value	180
Key References	181

Other Markers in the HLA Linkage Group

Pablo Rubinstein

I. Introduction	183
II. Genetic Considerations	185

III. Other Markers in the HLA Linkage Group	186
IV. Complement Components	187
V. Intracellular Enzymes	191
VI. Concluding Remarks	193
Selected References	194

INDEX 195

List of Contributors

Numbers in parentheses indicate the pages on which the authors' contributions begin.

FRITZ H. BACH, Immunobiology Research Center and Department of Medical Genetics, University of Wisconsin, Madison, Wisconsin 53706 (123)

H. CANTOR, Harvard Medical School/Farber Cancer Institute, Harvard University, Boston, Massachusetts 02115 (89)

MAX D. COOPER, Cellular Immunobiology Unit of the Tumor Institute, Departments of Pediatrics and Microbiology, and The Comprehensive Cancer Center, University of Alabama in Birmingham, Birmingham, Alabama 35294 (47)

ROBERT A. GOOD, Memorial Sloan–Kettering Cancer Center and Orthopedic Institute, Hospital for Joint Diseases, New York, New York 10021 (1)

SUDHIR GUPTA, Memorial Sloan–Kettering Cancer Center and Orthopedic Institute, Hospital for Joint Diseases, New York, New York 10021 (1)

RONALD B. HERBERMAN, Laboratory of Immunodiagnosis, National Cancer Institute, Bethesda, Maryland 20014 (73)

F. KISSMEYER-NIELSEN, Tissue-Typing Laboratory, University Hospital, DK-8000 Aarhus C, Denmark (99)

LORENZO MORETTA, Institute of Microbiology, University of Genova, 16132 Genova, Italy (47)

G. G. PERSIJN, Department of Immunohematology, University Medical Center, and Eurotransplant Foundation, Leiden, The Netherlands (161)

GORDON D. ROSS, Division of Rheumatology and Immunology, University of North Carolina Medical School, Chapel Hill, North Carolina 27514 (33)

PABLO RUBINSTEIN, The Lindsley F. Kimball Research Institute of the New York Blood Center, Inc., New York, New York 10021 (183)

L. P. RYDER, HLA and Disease Registry, Tissue-Typing Laboratory, State University Hospital of Copenhagen (Rigshospitalet), Blegdamsvej 9, DK-2100 Copenhagen Ø, Denmark (173)

DOLORES J. SCHENDEL, Institute for Immunology, University of Munich, Schillerstrasse 42, 0-8000 Munich-2, Federal Republic of Germany (143)

PAUL M. SONDEL,* The Immunobiology Research Center and Department of Medical Genetics, University of Wisconsin, Madison, Wisconsin 53706 (123)

JOHN D. STOBO, Section of Rheumatology and Clinical Immunology, Moffitt Hospital, University of California, San Francisco, California 94143 (55)

A. SVEJGAARD, HLA and Disease Registry, Tissue-Typing Laboratory, State University Hospital of Copenhagen (Rigshospitalet), Blegdamsvej 9, DK-2100, Copenhagen Ø, Denmark (173)

A. VAN LEEUWEN, Department of Immunohematology, University Medical Center, and Eurotransplant Foundation, Leiden, The Netherlands (113)

*Present address: Department of Pediatrics, CSC, 600 Highland Avenue, Madison, Wisconsin 53706.

J. J. VAN ROOD, Department of Immunohematology, University Medical Center, and Eurotransplant Foundation, Leiden, The Netherlands (113, 161)

ROBERT J. WINCHESTER, Memorial Sloan–Kettering Cancer Center and Orthopedic Institute, Hospital for Joint Diseases, New York, New York 10021 (1)

Preface

Two areas of immunobiology that have evoked great interest during the past several years concern themselves with definitions and characterizations of lymphoid subpopulations and with studies of the major histocompatibility complex (MHC). We have, in previous volumes, dealt with both these areas in a general manner; in this volume our intention has been to bring together in a more complete format information contributed by some of the leaders in these two areas.

The material presented will allow the nonspecialist in immunobiology and perhaps some specialists who are not directly working in one or both of these areas to gain a more thorough base of information that is required for adequate understanding and interpretation of data being published in the many journals dealing with immunobiology.

The first part of the volume includes a series of chapters dealing with present-day understanding of various subpopulations of cells involved in the immune system. The first chapter attempts to provide an overview to this problem, delving into the complexities inherent in subset definition and the methods available in that regard.

The next three chapters focus in greater detail on three techniques that have proved most valuable to the classification of cells, either by their cell surface phenotype or by their responsiveness to a series of different stimuli. Ross reviews the methods for detection of complement receptors and expression of these receptors on the surface of both normal and leukemic human lymphocytes. This area, i.e., defining cell subsets on the basis of which complement receptors they express, has made use of an increasing understanding of the complement system and has provided data that are most valuable. While pointing out that the exact function of complement receptors in immune response has not been elucidated, the author discusses the possible implications of complement synthesis by various cells involved in immune response and provides plausible models for correlating expression of these cell surface molecules with function.

Moretta and Cooper discuss their finding that different T-lymphocyte populations differentially express receptors for IgG or IgM. This observation, which has been widely used since description by these authors, is discussed not only with regard to the enumeration and isolation of T-cell subsets, but also with regard to the function of cells forming IgG or IgM rosettes and the clinical relevance of the subpopulations. Mitogens have long been used to activate T and other lymphocytes. The results discussed by Stobo demonstrate that differential responsiveness to the various mitogens can be used in delineating human lymphocyte differentiation and function. This area takes on all the more significance as the various products of cells activated with mitogens are used as "factors" influencing immune responsiveness. Stobo discusses these aspects of the problem and relates them to imbalances between the immunoregulatory cells.

The findings by several groups in 1975 relating to the existence of cytotoxic cells that preexist in the body, i.e., without overt antigenic stimulation, and referred to as natural killer (NK) cells, have led to a truly vast amount of effort to understand these cells and their importance in tumor surveillance. Herberman, who together with his colleagues, has been most active in this field, reviews NK cells and relates findings with those cells to antibody-dependent cell-mediated cytotoxicity (ADCC). Despite the rapid progress in this field, the review provides a solid framework to allow the reader to subsequently delve further into the current literature.

So much of our understanding of T-lymphocyte subpopulations relates to studies in mouse. In the last chapter of this section, Cantor provides an overview of those studies, primarily based on work with anti-Ly sera which has proved so useful for delineating T-cell subsets in that species. It seems very likely that a similar system will be defined in man; the material presented by Cantor may offer us some preview of what is and will be happening as the monoclonal anti-T-cell sera are further developed in man.

The second half of the volume deals with the major histocompatibility complex in man, HLA. This complex, which was first described in its relationship to serology of cell surface antigens and reactivity in the mixed leukocyte culture test, has taken a central place in two active areas of modern medicine: transplantation (including kidney and bone marrow as well as other organs) and disease associations. In the chapters presented, an attempt is made, first, to provide information regarding the methods of detection that are available to define antigens encoded by HLA genes and, second, to discuss some of the applications as they relate to transplantation and disease susceptibility.

Two major approaches have been taken for the definition of HLA encoded antigens: serology and T-lymphocyte reactivities. Thus, in the first chapter, Kissmeyer-Nielsen reviews the serology of the A, B, and C loci, antigens that are found on the surface of essentially all nucleated cells. In the second chapter, van Rood and van Leeuwen review the genetics and expression of the HLA-DR antigens that are found on the surface of cells of only a few tissues and which are thought to be the homologues of H-2 Ia antigens.

The next two chapters present a review of the methods that (a) employ "proliferative responses" in either mixed leukocyte cultures (MLCs) or primed LD typing (PLT) tests for measurement of antigens encoded largely in the HLA-D region, by Bach and Sondel, and (b) "cytotoxic responses," by Schendel, which in large measure relate to antigens of the HLA-A, -B, and -C loci, although it is not clear that the target antigens for cytotoxic T lymphocytes operative in these tests, i.e., the CD determinants, are identical to the serologically defined determinants of HLA-A, -B, and -C.

The area of HLA and graft survival has been one of the most intriguing and yet perplexing in this entire field. Whereas studies in HLA identical siblings provide the very strongest evidence showing that genes of the HLA complex are intimately involved in a very significant manner in determining whether a transplanted kidney will survive or not, it has been most difficult to find which of the HLA antigens, or perhaps combinations of antigens, must be "matched" between donor and recipient to insure good graft survival. van Rood and Persijn review this area both from the perspective of matching for the HLA-A, -B, and -C antigens, as well as matching for DR antigens.

Svejgaard and Ryder, who have headed the International HLA and Disease Registry, review the enormously important and popular area dealing with associations between HLA antigens and a variety of different diseases. The perspective that these authors have brought to this field is beautifully mirrored in their presentation and should provide the reader with the type of background necessary to evaluate the almost weekly reports that appear in the literature regarding the latest association. The final chapter in the volume, by Rubinstein, discusses other genetic markers in the HLA linkage group. This discussion is useful not only from the genetic point of view, but also for the reasons Rubinstein alludes to in his concluding remarks. A very fertile area for investigation exists as studies relate to these other markers.

We hope, and believe, that our choice of these two areas is most timely and that the presentations will provide the reader with an opportunity, at the very least, to develop an intellectual framework into which more detailed information can be fitted.

FRITZ H. BACH
ROBERT A. GOOD

Contents of Previous Volumes

Volume 1

Structure–Function Relations in the Lymphoid System
   Robert A. Good
The Immunoglobulins
   Richard Hong
Cellular Immunity
   H. Sherwood Lawrence
Transplantation Immunology
   Thomas E. Starzl and Charles W. Putnam
Immunological Tolerance
   A. C. Allison
Inflammation
   Michael T. Lamm and Chandler A. Stetson, Jr.
Fundamental Immunogenetics—Their Application to Histocompatibility
   Fritz H. Bach and Marilyn L. Bach
Humoral Amplification Systems in Inflammation
   Lawrence G. Hunsicker, Bruce U. Wintroub, and K. Frank Austen
Immunosuppression
   Eugene M. Lance
Tumor Immunology
   George Klein
Allergy
   L. M. Lichtenstein

Immunological Deficiency Disease
   Fred S. Rosen
SUBJECT INDEX

Volume 2

Bone Marrow Transplantation
   E. Donnall Thomas
Bone Marrow Transplantation for Aplasias and Leukemias
   G. Mathé, L. Schwarzenberg, N. Kiger, I. Florentin,
   O. Halle-Pannenko, and E. Garcia-Giralt
Bone Marrow and Thymus Transplants:
Cellular Engineering to Correct Primary Immunodeficiency
   Robert A. Good and Fritz H. Bach
Selective Immunotherapy with Transfer Factor
   H. Sherwood Lawrence
Transfer Factor
   Lynn E. Spitler, Alan S. Levin, and H. Hugh Fudenberg
Transfer Factor Therapy in Immunodeficiencies
   C. Griscelli
Immunological Surveillance: Pro and Con
   Richmond T. Prehn
Serology of Cancer
   Herbert F. Oettgen
The Role of Cell-Mediated Immunity in Control and
Growth of Tumors
   Karl Erik Hellström and Ingegerd Hellström
Experimental Models of Tumor Immunotherapy
   Jon R. Schmidtke and Richard L. Simmons
Graft versus Leukemia
   Mortimer M. Bortin
SUBJECT INDEX

Volume 3

Evaluation of the Immunoglobulins
   Richard Hong

Electrophoresis and Immunoelectrophoresis in the Evaluation of Homogeneous Immunoglobulin Components
  Edward C. Franklin
Serum Concentrations of IgG Subclasses
  Andreas Morell, Frantisek Skvaril, and Silvio Barandun
Imbalances of the κ/λ Ratio of Human Immunoglobulins
  Silvio Barandun, Frantisek Skvaril, and Andreas Morell
Metabolism of Immunoglobulins
  Thomas A. Waldmann and Warren Strober
Cell-Mediated Immunity: *In Vivo* Testing
  Carl M. Pinsky
Cellular Immunity: Antibody-Dependent Cytotoxicity (K-Cell Activity)
  Peter Perlmann
Short-Term ^{51}Cr-Release Tests for Direct Cell-Mediated Cytotoxicity: Methods, Clinical Uses, and Interpretations
  J. Wunderlich
Lymphocyte Transformation *in Vitro* in Response to Mitogens and Antigens
  Susanna Cunningham-Rundles, John A. Hansen, and Bo Dupont
Products of Activated Lymphocytes
  Ross E. Rocklin
Leukocyte Aggregation Test for Evaluating Cell-Mediated Immunity
  Baldwin H. Tom and Barry D. Kahan
The HLA System: Serologically Defined Antigens
  Ekkehard D. Albert
Mixed Leukocyte Cultures: A Cellular Approach to Histocompatibility Testing
  Fritz H. Bach
The Reticuloendothelial System
  W. F. Cunningham-Rundles
Assessment of Allergic States: IgE Methodology and the Measurement of Allergen-Specific IgG Antibody
  N. Franklin Adkinson, Jr., and Lawrence M. Lichtenstein
Autoantibodies in Hematological Disorders
  C. P. Engelfriet
Rheumatoid Factors in Human Disease
  Hugo E. Jasin and J. Donald Smiley
Antibodies to Nucleic Acids
  Norman Talal

Complement
  Harvey R. Colten and Chester A. Alper
Detection of Tumor-Associated Antigens in Plasma or Serum
  Morton K. Schwartz
Neutrophil Function
  Michael E. Miller
SUBJECT INDEX

Clinical Immunobiology

VOLUME 4

General Orientation of Human Lymphocyte Subpopulations[1]

SUDHIR GUPTA, ROBERT J. WINCHESTER,
and ROBERT A. GOOD

Memorial Sloan–Kettering Cancer Center and Orthopedic Institute, Hospital for Joint Diseases, New York, New York

I. Introduction	2
A. Background	2
B. Markers on the Cell Surface	3
C. Lymphocyte Populations	4
II. Cytoplasmic Immunoglobulin	5
III. Membrane Immunoglobulin	6
A. Ig Classes	6
B. Changes in Surface Ig	7
C. Methods and Technical Problems	8
IV. Ia System	9
A. Background	9
B. Methods of Detection	10
C. Cellular Distribution	11
V. Epstein–Barr Virus (EBV) Receptor	12
VI. Complement Receptors	13
VII. Receptors for Fc Region of Immunoglobulins	14
A. The IgG Fc Receptor	14
B. The IgM Fc Receptor	16

[1] Part of the work cited in this chapter is supported by grants from National Institute of Health CA-17404, CA-19267, CA-08748, CA-20499, CA-20107, AI-11843, NS-11457, AG-00541, Career Development Award A-11 00216, and funds for the advanced study of cancer and Judith Harris Selig Memorial Fund.

C. The IgA Fc Receptor	16
D. The IgE Fc Receptor	16
E. The IgD Fc Receptor	17
VIII. Enzymatic Markers	17
A. α-Napthyl Acetate Esterase	17
B. Acid Phosphatase	18
C. Terminal Deoxynucleotidyl Transferase (TdT)	18
IX. Receptors for Peanut Agglutinin	18
X. Erythrocyte Receptors	19
A. Receptors for SRBC	19
B. Receptors for Rhesus Monkey Erythrocytes	20
C. Receptors for Mouse Erythrocytes	21
D. Receptors for Macaca Monkey RBC	21
XI. Surface Antigens of Lymphocyte Subpopulations Defined by Monoclonal Antibodies	21
A. Background	21
B. Monoclonal Antibodies	23
C. Clinical Application of Monoclonal Antibodies	25
XII. Relationship between Tγ Cells and Monocytes	26
XIII. Distinction of Lymphocytes from Monocytes	28
XIV. The Third-Cell Population or Unclassified Lymphoid Cells	29
XV. Summary	30
References	30

I. Introduction

A. BACKGROUND

Rapid progress has been made in the last decade in defining the heterogeneity of lymphocytes with regard to morphology, cytochemistry, enzymatic markers, and surface receptors and/or antigens. This article will introduce the general approaches and some of the specific methods that are used to recognize distinct categories of lymphocytes, based on their differences in surface markers and antigens.

Both B and T lymphocytes are considered to originate from the multipotential hematopoietic stem cell, along with the other blood elements. The differentiation events that result in the functionally distinct lymphocyte lineages contribute to the diversity of lymphocyte populations as defined by surface markers. Furthermore, the common origin of lymphocytes and the other blood elements suggests the possibility that certain membrane components may occur on nonlymphoid cells that interfere with estimations of the lymphocyte populations. Under certain circumstances this can be a serious problem and considerable effort has been devoted to development of methods for identifying and separating out the nonlymphoid cells.

B. Markers on the Cell Surface

Two general types of determinants in the membrane that are used as lymphocyte population markers are antigens and receptors. A receptor is recognized by the specific ability to bind a particular labeled substance. Often the substance is attached to the surface of an erythrocyte, in which case the indication of the presence of a receptor is signaled by the formation of a rosette of erythrocytes about the central lymphocyte. Membrane antigens are detected by specific antibodies, using conventional immunological methods that have been modified for use on intact cells. Another method is now being developed which utilizes microchemical methodologies which define stages of differentiation. These are included as an example detection of differences in enzyme expression. More recently monoclonal antibodies prepared by the relatively new hybridoma technology have been developed which are improving definition of differentiation antigens on subpopulations of functionally distinct lymphocytes. This development is in an explosive stage based upon its apparent crucial revolutions of lymphocyte subsets in the mouse and it could be the basis for a complete revolution in cellular differentiation. Application of this approach to the analysis of immunodeficiency diseases and malignancies of the lymphoid systems has already begun.

A common characteristic of many of the methods used is that they analyze components on the surface membrane of living cells and can be modified so that viable cells are recoverable following the analysis. This results in three major areas of application of studies on lymphocytes surface markers. The first is analytic and involves the enumeration of specific lymphocyte populations, often with the objective of determining whether a patient has a particular lymphoproliferative disease or deficiency of cells as in immune deficiency. The second class of application is preparative and has as its objective the isolation for further analysis of a pure population of cells by virtue of the expression of a particular marker. A third class of application involves experiments on the immune response *in vitro* which take advantage of the fact that critical functional interactions of the lymphocytes in immune recognition and response occur through surface components. These experiments analyze cell function by alterations induced through manipulations of cell surface components.

In general, an analytic approach to lymphocyte classification requires an awareness of three problems. The first is a technical one and concerns performance of unambiguous measurement of the particular marker without interference from other receptors or components on the lymphocyte surface. The second is an experimental problem of defining the variety and quantifying the number of cells upon which a given marker is present in order to be able to make the proper inference concerning the type of lymphocyte population characterized by this marker. Finally in pathological states changes in the number of circulating cells or changes in the apparent properties of the cells with disease may not reflect functional abnormalities of the lymphocyte subpopulations in question.

C. Lymphocyte Populations

Lymphocytes may be divided into three major populations: B cells, T cells, and a third population of lymphoid cells which is neither T nor B. Each population may be further divided into subpopulations. The surface membrane of the typical B lymphocyte is characterized by certain well-defined molecules, such as readily detectable surface immunoglobulin and Ia molecules. In addition, receptors for Epstein–Barr virus and also receptors that bind to fragments of the C3 component of complement and receptors that bind to the Fc region of IgG, IgM, IgA, or IgD may be found on B lymphocytes. B lymphocytes comprise approximately 10–15% of peripheral blood lymphocytes.

T lymphocytes constitute the major population of peripheral blood lymphocytes, accounting for 80–85% of these cells. They are primarily recognized by a characteristic property of forming rosettes directly with a constituent present on the membrane of sheep erythrocytes (E rosettes). This property of E rosette formation is not shared by the typical B cell. A variable proportion of T cells also express receptors for the Fc region of IgG, IgM, IgA, IgE, or IgD. More recently, differentiation antigens on T cells have been recognized with immunologic reagents and T cells subpopulations may be identified by heteroantisera and monoclonal antibodies against these determinants prepared by hybridoma technique.

Lymphocytes having either B or T markers comprise 90–95% of all lymphocytes. The remaining lymphocytes may be recognized in peripheral blood by the fact that they lack both Ig determinants and ability to form E rosettes. Such cells are said to constitute a third or null population of lymphoid cells. Since this population contains precursor cells of both lymphoid and nonlymphoid cell lineage, we prefer to refer to them as "unclassified" lymphoid cells. There is little question that they represent a most heterogeneous population that contains a small population of precursor of monocytes, committed precursors of granulocyte–monocyte lineage, precursors of eosinophils and probably basophils, precursors of other hematopoietic cells, and even a few stem cells with multipotentiality. In addition to these small populations the null lymphocytes also contain a population of cells that may be important in antibody-dependent cytotoxicity and other functions in the immunological defense.

The following sections will review markers in common use that distinguish populations and subpopulations of lymphocytes.

II. Cytoplasmic Immunoglobulin

The earliest presently identifiable cell of the B cell lineage is the so-called pre-B cell. These cells are identified by the presence of intracytoplasmic immunoglobulin, but they lack surface immunoglobulin. According to morphologic and kinetic studies, pre-B cells appear to be divisible into two classes. The large pre-B cell (~ 17 μm) has a deeply indented or convoluted nucleus and represents cells undergoing rapid proliferation. The small pre-B cell (~ 9 μm) has a morphology similar to that of surface IgM positive B cells, but lack surface IgM, contain cytoplasmic IgM, and are slowly dividing cells. A subpopulation of pre-B cells and cells from certain patients with pre-B cell leukemia have Ia-like antigen at their surface. Pre-B cells lack Fc receptors for immunoglobulin but appear to have Epstein–Barr (EB) virus receptors. Thus cell lines have been made of pre-B cells from bone marrow of certain patients with X-lined infantile agammaglobulinemia by exposing the cells to EB virus *in vitro*. Pre-B cells outnumber surface IgM-positive B cells in fetal liver up to the thirteenth week of gestation. In postnatal life pre-B cells are almost exclusively restricted to bone marrow ($\sim 0.8\%$ of total mononuclear cells). Pre-B cells are present in normal proportions in the bone marrow from patients with

X-linked infantile agammaglobulinemia (Burton's disease). Plasma cells also contain intracytoplasmic immunoglobulin; however, they differ from pre-B cells in that they are specialized to synthesize and secrete any one of the immunoglobulins with descrete heavy chains. The Ig secreted is generally identical to the Ig present on the surface of the B lymphocytes prior to events involved in the terminal stage of differentiation. Almost all pre-B cells contain only cytoplasmic IgM. By *in vitro* manipulations, it has not been possible to induce pre-B cells to differentiate into mature B cells. Pre-B cell lines cultured from patients with X-linked agammaglobulinemia appear to include precursor cells that possess receptors for EBV, but no Ig chains or molecules. Pre-B cells have cytoplasmic μ heavy chain, but do not synthesize light chains and lack surface IgM. Another kind of pre-B cells grown from these patients contains cytoplasmic IgM having both light and heavy chains, but no surface Ig. Each of these cell types has receptors for EB virus. They are more readily obtained from the marrow of patients with X-linked infantile agammaglobulinemia than from bone marrow of normals because cultures of normal marrow readily show classical B cells that are lacking in patients with X-linked agammaglobulinemia and in the presence of EB virus they overgrow the cultures.

III. Membrane Immunoglobulin

Membrane immunoglobulin (MIg) is a component expressed only on lymphocytes, almost certainly only on cells of the B cell population. The MIg molecules act as receptors for recognition of antigen. The antibody present on the surface of individual B cells is homogeneous in its specificity for antigen. The MIg represents antibodies of the specificity that will ultimately be synthesized by the plasma cell which is derived from the lymphocyte following antigen-induced terminal differentiation.

A. Ig Classes

The striking feature about MIg is that the number of cells bearing each of the different Ig classes does not parallel the quantity of the individual Ig in serum. Thus, while IgG and IgA are major serum Igs, only a very few circulating B lymphocytes have IgG or IgA as a dominant surface Ig. Rather, IgM plus IgD comprise the predominant cell surface Ig on B lymphocytes that are present in peripheral blood. Approximately two-thirds of B lymphocytes bearing Ig at their surface express both IgM and IgD, and the remaining one-third consists of cells expressing only IgM or IgD on the surface. In terms of the sequence of appearance of Ig, the consensus is that surface IgM is the Ig that first become apparent on B lymphocytes. This stage is followed by cells that express both IgD and IgM on their surface. Studies have demonstrated that both the IgM and IgD on the surface of individual B cells have the same antibody-combining sites. Thus the cells appear to express the product of the same gene coding for the antibody-combining site. An interesting restriction in Ig expression is evident in that a single lymphocyte expresses only one or the other light chains, κ or λ, but not both. Rapid progress is being made to unravel the details of gene action in antibody and Ig development applying rapidly developing tools of molecular biology.

B. Changes in Surface Ig

The transition of B lymphocytes from a precursor cell through the sequence of surface IgM and IgM plus IgD is independent of antigen exposure. This switch is of considerable interest, since it appears to influence, and perhaps determine, the type of immune response that will result from contact with antigen. It is now considered likely that cells with only IgM as the only surface Ig are more easily induced to give a response resulting in tolerance. When IgD appears at the surface tolerance is difficult to induce. Evidence now exists that the cells bearing surface IgM plus IgD give rise to the IgM-producing plasma cells characteristically developed during primary immune response. The secondary immune response is characterized by an elevated level of plasma cells and the cells that develop from this stimulus produce intracellular IgG or IgA.

The process whereby cells bearing surface Ig synthesize intracellular Ig is complicated because it is difficult to identify to what extent Ig present on the surface is intracellular Ig in the process of being transported out of the cell, and to what extent it is intrinsic membrane Ig. Nevertheless, generally very little or no surface IgG is detectable on the cell surface of plasma cells engaged in IgG synthesis. In newborns many of the B cells in the peripheral blood contain both IgM and

IgD and a considerable population may possess three different surface Ig, e.g., IgM + IgD + IgG or IgM + IgD + IgA. Similarly, such a high frequency of cells bearing double or triple Ig markers is seen in the peripheral blood B cells of patients with either common variable immunodeficiency or patients with selective absence of IgA. This high frequency of double or triple surface Ig is taken as a sign of immaturity of the B lymphocytes in these conditions.

C. Methods and Technical Problems

The preferred method to demonstrate surface Ig is direct immunofluorescence microscopy. The results of this method are in general agreement with immunoprecipitation analyses based on radiolabeled cell surface components and with analyses based on mixed hemaglutination. Cytotoxic methods of detecting antibody binding to B cells have proved to be difficult to perform reliably and have been used relatively little. The technique of immunofluorescence involves the use of antibodies specific for κ or λ or for the light chain determinants found on Fab fragments of IgG. Detection of the binding of the antibody tagged with a fluorochrome requires the use of intense illumination provided by an incident illumination device. The reference section contains articles that provide details of these methodologies.

A technical problem that requires special comment is the potential for interference caused by the presence of the IgG Fc receptor on certain B or T cells. Under certain conditions this receptor can bind either serum IgG or immune complexes made by an anti-IgG antibody and minute amounts of free IgG present in the cell supernatant. This results in the detection of this Ig by the fluorescent staining reaction. Alternatively, any aggregated or complexed fluorescent reagent will also directly bind the cell via the Fc receptor. These types of interference are especially subtle and have caused confusion regarding the number of IgG molecules on the lymphocyte that possess IgG on the surface. The staining reaction in this instance depends on the presence of anti-IgG antibodies and is abolished by appropriate specificity controls involving selective removal of antibodies to IgG from the cells, using latex-labeled cells, incubation of cells for several hours at 37°C, additional washing steps, and the use of $F(ab')_2$ fragments instead of intact IgG antibodies as the reagent antibodies in examining for cells bearing surface Ig.

Another technical aspect is that a distinction must be made between intracellular and cell surface Ig. Although immunofluorescence methods are used in both determinations, critical differences are of importance. Intracellular Ig is performed on dead or fixed cells that do not have the capacity to exercise the semipermeable property of the membrane, and under which circumstances the reagent antiserum has access to the cytoplasmic Ig. The quantity of Ig present on the cell surface is small compared to that in the cell interior, and thus the surface Ig does not interfere significantly with the intracellular determination. By contrast, the cell surface Ig requires that staining be made on viable cells with an intact membrane, and because the concentration of Ig on the surface is an order of magnitude less, special epiillumination procedures are required for visualization of fluorescence demonstrating the Ig at the cell surface.

Differentiation of B lymphocytes into antibody-secreting cells can also be quantified by estimating the formation of plaques on an appropriately labeled layer of erythrocytes. The erythrocyte target can have a hapten or antigen coupled to the surface that is recognized by antibodies secreted by the lymphocytes. The antibody-coated erythrocytes are then lysed by the addition of complement.

Methods designed to yield purified preparations of B lymphocytes, or cells depleted of B lymphocytes, primarily involve either the sorting of cells stained by fluorescent antibodies with a fluorescence-activated cell sorter or mechanical entrapment of Ig-bearing cells on anti-Ig-coated columns or the use of centrifugation methodology after rosetting with erythrocytes coated with anti-Ig.

IV. Ia System

A. BACKGROUND

There are two molecular systems, each composed of two polypeptide chains, that are products of major histocompatibility complex genes and are expressed on the cell surface membrane. One of these is the B_2-microglobulin-associated system that comprises the classic HLA antigens, HLA-A, -B, and -C. These antigens have a 45,000-dalton chain that, through apparent gene duplication, is coded for at three loci, *A*, *B*, or *C*, and which are highly polymorphic. This system is expressed on essentially all nucleated cells, including both T and B cells.

In addition, there is a second bimolecular system that in view of its structural homologies with the murine Ia system is designated Ia-like, or for simplicity Ia, when it is clear that the human situation is being referred to. The Ia molecule is composed of two chains: a 28,000-dalton light chain and a heavy chain approximately of 34,000–37,000 daltons. This system is selectively expressed on the surface of most B cells, but not on the vast majority of T lymphocytes. The Ia determinants represent a differentiation alloantigen of particular significance both in terms of cellular expression and in expression of particular alleles. It appears likely that there are multiple loci governing the synthesis of the relevant chains, but the genetic fine structure has not been definitively resolved and is the subject of much current investigation.

B. Methods of Detection

Three types of antisera are used to recognize Ia or Ia-like determinants. One type is a human serum reagent where an immunization with a foreign Ia histocompatibility determinant has occurred either as a consequence of pregnancy or transplantation of cells of tissues. These alloantisera are used in indirect fluorescence or cytotoxicity assays. The drawback of the alloantisera is the necessity of ascertaining that the individual to be tested expresses the appropriate allele.

The second approach is the use of a heteroantiserum raised against the Ia molecules from human B lymphocytes; here either lymphoid cell lines or leukemia cells are used to assure an adequate supply of antigen. Ia molecules comprise nearly 10% of the membrane glycoproteins in certain lymphoid cell lines and are readily isolated from the cell membrane by detergent solubilization followed by gel filtration and gel electrophoresis. The simplicity of producing a potent heteroantiserum that can be used in direct fluorescence obviates the need to select proper alloantiserum and avoids use of indirect assays. This approach has greatly facilitated the use of Ia system as a B lymphocyte marker.

The third, a more recent approach is to use monoclonal antibody against "Ia-like" determinants. When such monoclonal antibodies with a variety of "Ia" specificities become available, the other two systems will almost certainly be replaced by this technique.

C. Cellular Distribution

1. Ia Antigens on Cells of B Lymphocyte Lineage

Of particular concern is the question of whether Ia determinants on a lymphocyte are indicative that the cell is of the B lineage. Several lines of evidence strongly support an affirmative answer to this question and illustrate the utility of the Ia molecules as B cell markers. The first is that all cells bearing surface IgM or IgD express Ia, as shown in experiments using double-labeling technique. The second is that the average number of cells that exceeds the number of B cells recognized by IgM and IgD by approximately 25–35%. $Ig^- Ia^+$ cells are not found in patients with the X-linked infantile agammaglobulinemia; and furthermore, in normal individuals the majority of the $Ig^- Ia^+$ lymphocytes express complement receptors, implying a stage of primarily within the B lineage, presumably reflecting a stage of differentiation where surface Ig is difficult to recognize. It has recently been reported that a subpopulation of normal and malignant pre-B cells expresses Ia antigens.

In the terminal stage of normal and malignant B cell differentiation, the Ia antigens are no longer expressed on the cell surface, and most plasma cells lack Ia determinants. Of interest in this regard is the presence of abundant surface Ia on B cells that have been stimulated by pokeweed mitogen. This finding implies that the signal provided by the lectin induces differentiation to plasma cells but involves changes in cell surface that reflect characteristics of proliferating cells.

2. Ia Antigens on Monocytes

Because circulating monocytes also have Ia determinants until late in the differentiation sequence, it is apparent that Ia-bearing monocytes must be distinguished from lymphocytes. It is also possible that rare hematopoietic progenitors or myeloblasts bearing Ia determinants are present in detectable numbers in peripheral blood.

3. Ia Antigens on T Cells

The problem of Ia determinants on lymphocytes that form E rosettes requires comment. Of lymphocytes isolated by the property of E rosette formation, 1–4% bear readily detectable Ia antigens. A variable proportion of these cells bear surface Ig, and some appear to represent B cells that presumably have antibody receptors for determinants on sheep erythrocytes. Of much greater significance is accumulating evidence that E rosette-forming cells which do not have any B cell markers have definitely recognizable Ia determinants. The nature of these cells and the nature of the Ia molecules on them are matters of great current interest. Stimulation of T cells by mitogens and in mixed lymphocyte cultures enhances the expression of Ia molecules at their surface and results in a larger number of E rosette-forming cells bearing Ia determinants. The nature of this subpopulation of T cells remains to be determined.

4. Ia Antigens on Nonlymphoid Cells

The picture that is emerging of the Ia system is that the expression of the Ia molecule on the surface membrane of either normal or malignant cells is an event primarily dependent on the differentiation state of the cell. Second, the Ia system is predominantly expressed on cells originating from the hematopoietic–lymphoid system. Among nonlymphoid cells, in the erythroid and granulocyte lineages, only the progenitor cells capable of colony formation and the earliest morphologically recognizable level of differentiating cells bear Ia determinants. Thus, in the granulocyte lineage the Ia molecules are lost at the level of the promyelocyte. The function of the Ia system on these cells, not apparently involved in immune functions, may relate to control of cell proliferation in the bone marrow. Ia antigen is also expressed on the Langerhans cells of the skin and umbilical vein.

V. Epstein–Barr Virus (EBV) Receptor

The EB virus is lymphotropic in man. EB virus binds to the surface of some B cell blasts of lymphoid cell lines in long-term culture but apparently does not bind to cells of T cell lines. Thymocytes and resting or activated T cells also lack receptors for EBV. EBV receptor is present on virtually all B lymphocyte and also on a subpopulation of the third lymphoid cell population. These cells may be precursors for B lymphocytes. The closely linked disappearance and reappearance of EBV receptors and complement receptors in a cell line originally isolated from a Burkitt lymphoma line strongly suggest that these two receptors are either identical or closely linked constituents of the cell membrane. The apparent restriction of EBV binding sites to B lymphocytes implies that B lymphocytes are a target for *in vivo* transformation by EBV.

VI. Complement Receptors

Lymphocyte express membrane receptors for C3b, C4d (immune adherence receptor), C3d, C1q, and possibly factor B of the alternative pathway of the complement system. Two different types of C receptors known as CR_1 (C4b) and CR_2 (C3d) on the surface of lymphocytes have been extensively studied. These two C receptors are structurally distinct and are located on separate molecules present on the lymphocyte membrane. Three different C components bind to C receptors; C4, C3, and C5. These three proteins share a common structure that allows binding to CR_1-type receptors. In addition, C3 contains two other receptor binding sites that bind C3 to either CR_2-type or CR_3-type receptors. The binding sites in C3 for CR_3 attachment are distinct from both the CR_1 and CR_2 binding sites and are believed to be located between the c and d regions of C3 that may contain the small C3e fragment. The C3b molecule binds to either the CR_1 or CR_3 binding sites but leaves the CR_2 site that binds to the C3d molecule. The C4b molecule resembles C3b in that it has a site for attachment to CR_1. However, enzymatic breakdown of C4b by plasma-protein destroys the CR_1 binding site without exposing hidden binding sites for either CR_2 or CR_3.

Peripheral blood lymphocytes are subdivided into two subpopulations with respect to complement receptors. One of these is characterized by having only CR_1 and the other by having both CR_1 and CR_2. This latter population is essentially identical to the classic B cells with surface Ig and Ia-like antigens. The lymphocytes bearing only CR_1 lack surface Ig and are further divided between those considered to belong to the B cell lineage because they possess readily demonstrable Ia-like antigen. The other cells probably belong to the T cell lineage and they lack Ia antigens but possess E rosette receptors. Essentially, all lymphocytes with CR_1, CR_2 receptors have Fc receptors; however, the reverse does not appear to be true. Fetal thymocytes have also been shown to bear C receptors; however, it is not known whether the receptors they have are CR_1 or CR_2 or both.

C1q receptors are present on both T and B lymphocytes. This receptor is trypsin sensitive but resistant to treatment with neuraminidase or DNase. The finding that C1q binds to T lymphocytes and Raji cells that lack membrane-bound Ig, and also to Daudi cells that are devoid of detectable amounts of B_2-microglobulin, suggests that the C1q receptor is distinct from the other membrane markers. The biologic significance of the C1q receptor is unknown. It is possible that this receptor binds activated C1 which in turn activates the complement sequence and generates a change of cell activity.

VII. Receptors for Fc Region of Immunoglobulins

The lymphocyte membrane contains receptors for the Fc region of immunoglobulin.

A. THE IgG Fc RECEPTOR

Receptors that react with the Fc region of IgG immunoglobulin are of particular interest because, although they are expressed on a minority of peripheral blood lymphocytes, their occurrence is not restricted to one lymphocyte lineage. The IgG Fc receptor has been demonstrated on the vast majority of B cells, some of the third population cells, and on a minor population of T cells, termed Tγ.

To a certain extent divergent reports in the literature regarding the presence or the absence of IgG Fc receptors on particular lymphocyte types have made this a relatively confusing area. One reason for this is that much variation exists in the extent of binding that can be achieved with a particular Fc receptor detection system for the receptors on a particular lymphocyte subpopulation. This issue will be discussed below. It reflects an underlying heterogeneity for the reactivity of Fc receptors on T cells and third-population lymphocytes while those on B lymphocytes are more constant.

The function of the IgG Fc receptor on most cells is still not well understood. However, on a subpopulation of cells that includes the third population and Tγ cells, Fc receptors are essential for antibody-dependent cell-mediated cytotoxicity.

To determine the relationship of Fc receptors to the lymphocyte subpopulations, a sequence of isolation and identification is necessary for recognition of B cells, T cells, and third-population cells. One strategy is to fractionate the lymphocyte population initially according to the presence or the absence of capacity to form stable rosettes with sheep erythrocytes. This procedure involves use of a relatively delicate rosette interaction. It has an inherent hazard of selecting only T lymphocytes that form the most stable rosettes. Thus the residual non-T population is contaminated with T cells that have lower avidity for sheep erythrocytes. Thus care is necessary to achieve meaningful results. A second step is the identification of the Ia-bearing cells in the fraction that does not form rosettes with sheep erythrocytes because Ia antisera inhibit IgG Fc receptors, minimal quantities of $F(ab')_2$ reagents must be used to define cells of the B lineage so as not to interfere with subsequent assays.

Evidence now indicates that two types of IgG Fc receptor are distinguishable by particular test systems. One is associated with T cells and the other with B cells.

At least six different Fc receptor test systems have been employed on separated and well-characterized lymphocyte populations. A wide variation was observed when these were used to detect IgG Fc receptors. For example, according to one method used, the number of Ia^+ cells expressing Fc receptors varied from 3 to 90%, of T cells from 1 to 11%, and third populations from 42 to 73%. It is apparent that the Fc receptors on B cells were best demonstrated in certain system which have reduced reactivity with T cells. By contrast other sytems, such as the EA rosette system with human anti-Rh antibodies, the reaction was preferential for T cells and Ia-negative non-T cells.

Underlying these reproducible variations that appear to relate to qualitative factors in the nature of the immune complex being used for detection is inherent change in reactivity of the Fc receptor with temperature. For example, at 4°C native 7 S IgG as well as purified Fc fragments bind strongly to the IgG Fc receptors, particularly as this is expressed on T cells. Thus these may be several different functions for Fc receptors and they may occur in more than one molecular form. It appears further that IgG Fc receptor expression is influenced by the functional state of the lymphocyte itself.

The IgG Fc receptor on Tγ cells may be modulated when the Tγ cells interact *in vitro* with insoluble immune complexes (e.g., antibody-coated OXRBC). During this process, IgG Fc receptors are lost from a subpopulation of Tγ cells and a proportion of these cells now express IgM Fc receptor.

B. THE IgM Fc RECEPTOR

Receptors for the Fc region of IgM have been found on B cells, on third population cells, and on T cells. They occur on a major subpopulation of T cells which lacks IgG Fc receptors. This subpopulation is termed Tμ. There is a small population of T cells that expresses receptors for both IgM Fc and IgG Fc. The B cell population is heterogeneous with respect to the presence of the IgM Fc receptor. This receptor is expressed particularly well on B cells from lymphoid organs and on leukemic B cells.

The IgM Fc receptor is normally detected by rosette assays using anti-erythrocyte antibodies of the IgM class to sensitize the erythrocytes. Inhibition studies using soluble IgM or IgM Fc fragments, however, illustrate that other methods will be possible. The binding site for IgM Fc on T cells receptor is to monomeric or pentameric IgM Fc.

C. THE IgA Fc RECEPTOR

Receptors for the Fc region of IgA have been found on T, B, or third population lymphoid cells. The receptor is present on a subpopulation of both normal or leukemic lymphocytes, Occasionally we have observed a small population of T lymphocytes bearing receptors for the Fc region of all three immunoglobulins, IgM, IgG, and IgA simultaneously. The role of IgA receptor on T or B cell subpopulations with IgA Fc receptor is not understood at present. IgA Fc receptor is also present on the surface of human polymorphonuclear neutrophils but is absent from monocytes and eosinophils.

The IgA Fc receptor is detected by a rosette assay which employs either anti-OXRBC antibody of IgA class to sensitized OXRBC or TNP-coated OXRBC treated with a mouse IgA myeloma (MOPC-315) that has anti-TNP specificity.

D. THE IgE Fc RECEPTOR

The IgE Fc receptors also exist on the surface of a very small population of both T and B lymphocytes. The role of IgE Fc on a subpopulation of T or B cells with IgE Fc receptor is not known. However, in animal systems it has been suggested that T cells with IgE Fc receptor (Tε) could play a helper role in IgE-specific immune response. Furthermore, when the level of IgE is high in serum or medium to which the cells are exposed, it results in an increase in Tε cells. This finding is consonant with our observation that increased numbers of Tε cells are present in the blood of patients with hyperimmunoglobulinemia E syndrome.

The IgE Fc receptor is detected by rosette assay in which IgE myeloma-coated RBC are used. IgE Fc receptor is present on some eosinophils but is absent on neutrophils and monocytes.

E. The IgD Fc Receptor

It is only very recently that a receptor for the Fc region of IgD has been demonstrated on a subpopulation of both T and non-T lymphocytes. Latex particles coated with IgD have been utilized to detect this receptor. The significance of this receptor, like that of other Fc receptors on lymphocytes, is unknown.

The two subpopulations of T cells with IgM Fc (Tμ) or IgG Fc (Tγ) receptor have been extensively studied for morphological, enzymatic, and functional characteristics and will be discussed in detail elsewhere in this volume.

VIII. Enzymatic Markers

A. α-Napthyl Acetate Esterase

The histochemical demonstration of nonspecific α-napthyl acetate esterase (ANAE) activity in monocytes is useful for identification of these cells in mixed mononuclear cell suspensions. Recently, ANAE activity has been demonstrated to be present also in human peripheral blood T cells and certain mitogen-stimulated T lymphocytes. The percentage of sheep red blood cell (SRBC) rosette-forming T cells and ANAE-positive lymphocytes is nearly comparable in the peripheral blood. However, a distinctive staining pattern characterizes the T lymphocytes and monocytes that stain with ANAE. Discrepancies from this point of view have been observed in certain tissues, e.g., spleen and thymus. Fewer thymocytes demonstrated ANAE activity than were found rosetting with SRBC. In spleen ANAE activity is present in non-T cells as well.

B. ACID PHOSPHATASE

Acid phosphatase, a hydrolytic enzyme, is present in various human tissues such as liver, prostate, and the cells of the hematopoietic system. Acid phosphatase staining, however, appears to have some specificity for thymus-related cells. This enzyme is found in a patchy paranuclear (Golgi) distribution. Acid phosphatase activity has been described in malignant cells of some T cells leukemias. The latter is tartrate-resistant and appears to be characteristic of abnormal cells from patients with hairy cell leukemia. However, occasionally cells from other lymphoproliferative disorders, such as prolymphocytic leukemia, lymphosarcoma cell leukemia, and Sezary syndrome may also have tartrate-resistant acid phosphatase.

C. TERMINAL DEOXYNUCLEOTIDYL TRANSFERASE (TdT)

Terminal deoxynucleotidyl transferase is an unusual DNA polymerase that does not use template information to synthesize new strands of DNA. The enzyme TdT may be used as a lymphoid cell marker. Originally TdT was considered to be restricted to cells in the thymus, but later TdT was demonstrated in bone marrow and human tonsils. TdT has been reported to be present in the cells of patients with acute lymphoblastic leukemia. The enzyme can be used as a marker for prothymocytes. It has, however, recently been shown that leukemic blasts from certain patients with pre-B cell leukemia and those from acute B cell leukemia may contain large amounts of TdT activity. Therefore, it is apparent that TdT cannot be taken as a marker exclusive for pre-T cells and that this enzyme may be present on precursors of several other hematopoietic cells.

IX. Receptors for Peanut Agglutinin

Receptors for peanut agglutinin appear to be a useful marker for identifying cells that are at a very early stage in the T cell differentiation. However, this receptor is not confined to cells of T cell lineage. The binding sites for the peanut lectin are present on cells from Burkitt Lymphoma (B cell lineage) as well as cells of acute myeloid leukemia.

X. Erythrocyte Receptors

A. Receptors for SRBC

The property of forming rosettes with sheep erythrocytes is an extremely useful marker of lymphocytes within the T lineage. If the lymphocytes with definite B cell markers are excluded, 90–95% of the residual lymphocytes form E rosettes. This figure can be brought toward 100% if the lymphocytes are first exposed to neuraminidase. Reciprocally, the vast preponderance of B lymphocytes do not form rosettes with sheep erythrocytes, even after neuraminidase treatment. Chronic lymphatic leukemia lymphocytes of the B variety serve as prototypes of B lymphocyte in that they do not form E rosettes under any condition of reaction, including following exposure to neuraminidase. Excluded from this discussion is the occasional B lymphocyte which has Ig receptors that bind specifically to determinants such as heterophil antigens that are present on SRBC. Chronic lymphatic leukemias of this variety occur and can be recognized by blockade of the receptor by anti-Ig.

The E rosette receptor is relatively weaker than complement or IgG Fc receptors detected by rosette formation. The strength of the interaction is enhanced by the addition of serum or by treatment of the erythrocyte by reducing agents or neuraminidase. The formation of rosettes is aided by gentle centrifugation and incubation at 4°C. Gentle resuspension is essential to permit estimation of the maximum number of E rosette-positive lymphocytes.

An important property of the E rosette is that the lymphocyte receptors for the sheep cell are of varying net avidity. Certain lymphocytes have relatively stronger binding of SRBC that occurs rapidly and at warmer temperatures. Cells with this property include a portion of the blood lymphocytes, the majority of thymocytes, and some lymphocytes found in pathological situations, for example, in the joint fluids of patients with rheumatoid arthritis. No definite pathogenic interpretation should be placed on the finding of these cells in view of the difficulty of obtaining proper control populations. Stimulation of the lymphocytes by lectins or by allogeneic cells also yields lymphocytes with an augmented ability to form rosettes.

Other lymphocytes are characterized by weaker rosette formation. These pose a particular problem because relatively slight variations in technique, e.g., variations in method used to resuspend the cells, yield different results. Thus values for E rosettes may very considerably from laboratory to laboratory. The consequences of this characteristic are significant because of the number of cells estimated to be in the "third," or "residual," population. The use of serum in the rosette reaction or modification of the erythrocyte surface such as with neuraminidase treatment stabilizes the rosettes.

Cells that have IgG Fc receptors but lack B cell markers, e.g., Ia and the Tγ cells, are the best examples of cell that form low affinity rosettes. As mentioned earlier, the identical pattern of Fc receptor reactivity in binding avidity, functional activity, as well as the effect of neuraminidase digestion are characteristic of cells in the third population that do not form E rosettes. Such third-population cells may actually be cells of T lineage. However, they are characterized by extremely weak or nonexistent E rosette binding. The limited avidity for E rosettes, in general, that characterizes these cells has resulted in conflicting reports in the literature regarding the occurrence of various Fc receptor activities in both the T and third population of lymphoid cells.

In summary, the E rosette phenomenon, because of its biological significance as a T cell marker, simplicity of assay, and the availability of the reagents, will remain an important means of enumerating T cells. However, progressively, it will be supplemented by or even replaced by monoclonal antibodies that identify surface antigens characteristic of all T cells.

B. Receptors for Rhesus Monkey Erythrocytes

Rhesus monkey RBC form spontaneous rosettes with a large population of peripheral blood lymphocytes and thymocytes. Indeed, in lymphocytes from normal adults, a linear correlation exists between the percentages of rosette-forming cells with rhesus monkey RBC and with SRBC. These observations suggest that this marker is present on T cells. However, it has been observed that rhesus monkey RBC also form spontaneous rosettes with B cells from certain patients with chronic lymphocytic leukemia and with third-population lymphoid cells from healthy controls.

C. Receptors for Mouse Erythrocytes

Mouse red blood cells (MRBC) form spontaneous rosettes with a subpopulation of B lymphocytes. Approximately 7–8% of peripheral blood lymphocytes form rosettes with MRBC. MRBC bind to most, but not exclusively all, of the B cells that have surface IgM. MRBC bind more avidly to relatively immature B cells. The most important use of this marker has been in diagnosis of chronic lymphocytic leukemia (CLL). CLL B cells have almost undetectable or very faint surface Ig, but are MRBC receptor positive. This marker assists in differentiating B cell CLL from B cell lymphoma in leukemic phase, lymphosarcoma cell leukemia. In the latter disease, MRBC do not bind to the malignant B cells.

The binding between B cells and MRBC is weak, requiring that MRBC be used no later than 2 days after bleeding. Therefore, this technique is not very effective for separating large numbers of B cells or B cell subpopulations.

D. Receptors for Macaca Monkey RBC

Macaca speciosa monkey RBC form spontaneous rosettes with human B cells and do not form rosettes with T lymphocytes. The binding with B lymphocyte is independent of IgG Fc, C3b, or C3d receptors.

XI. Surface Antigens of Lymphocyte Subpopulations Defined by Monoclonal Antibodies

A. Background

Investigations over the past 20 years have revealed that lymphocyte differentiation in the mouse is accompanied by a series of cell surface antigenic changes on the T lymphocytes which reflect distinct stages of differentiation and ultimately make it possible to identify distinct subpopulations of T lymphocytes that are specialized for certain func-

TABLE I
MONOCLONAL ANTIBODIES DEFINING DIFFERENTIATION
ANTIGENS OF HUMAN T LYMPHOCYTES

Antigens	Cell type expressing differentiation antigens
T10+	Early thymocyte
T10+	
T9+	
T10+	Common thymocyte
T6+	
T4+	
T5+	
T10+	Mature thymocyte
T1+	
T3+	
T4+	
T10+	Mature thymocyte
T1+	
T3+	
T5+	
T1+	Inducer/helper T lymphocyte
T3+	
T4+	
T1+	Suppressor/cytotoxic T lymphocyte
T3+	
T5+	

tions. Figure 1 illustrates these stages of differentiation for the prototype murine species. Investigations by Schlossman and his colleagues using the hybridoma technique to develop monoclonal antibodies against human thymocytes have shown that this goal can be achieved for human T lymphocytes. It seems certain that markers of distinct differentiation stages and ultimately distinct sets of B lymphocytes and perhaps even distinct sets of monocytes will be defined in the same way. Thus far at least 10 monoclonal antibodies have been developed by the hybridoma technique by Schlossman and his colleagues against human thymocytes and T lymphocytes. Some of these antibodies are already being made available through commercial sources. These antibodies are listed in Table I and the progress already made in identifying stages of human T cell differentiation is also summarized in this table. As can be seen in the table, certain of these antibodies permit recognition of early thymocytes, another constellation of antigens per-

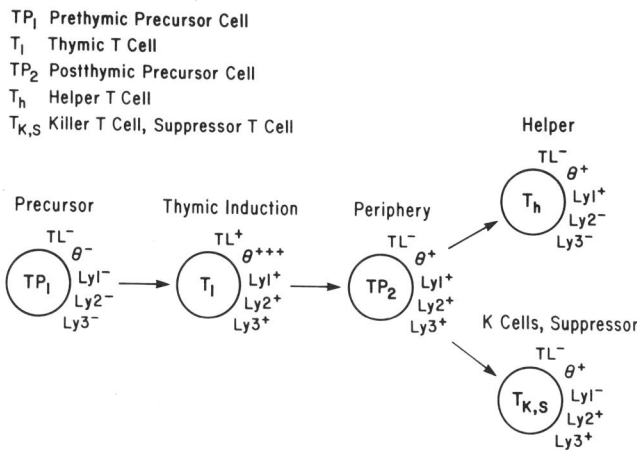

Fig. 1. Differentiation surface antigens on subpopulations of T cells in mouse.

mits definition of common thymocytes, still another of mature thymocytes, and a clear bifurcation to populations that contain functionally distinct helper/inducer and suppressor/cytotoxic cells can be identified. Finally, the functionally distinct subpopulations of peripheral T cells can also be distinguished by the appropriate antibodies that recognize cell surface antigenic characteristics.

B. Monoclonal Antibodies

The first clear designation of functionally distinct subpopulations in humans occurred when Evans and associates prepared a heteroantibody in rabbit called anti-TH2 which defined a subset of thymus and peripheral T lymphocytes. This subset contained T cells capable of exercising cytotoxic and suppressor activities. By contrast, peripheral and mature thymic T lymphocytes which did not bear this antigen contained the population of T cells capable of exercising helper T cell functions. Using hybridoma technique Reinherz and Schlossman (1980) have identified monoclonal antibodies designated anti-T9 and anti-T10 that can recognize antigens designated T9 and T10 that identify thymocytes at an early stage of differentiation. The common thymocyte was found to have an antigen designated T6 which is a likely candidate for the human equivalent of the TL antigen. Common thymocytes retain T10 antigen present on early thymocytes, but T9 antigen disappears from the surface of common thymocytes. In addition, common thymocytes express T4 and T5 antigens that are present on mature thymocytes and peripheral T cells. Mature thymocytes and peripheral T cells, in addition, express T1 antigen. T10 antigen disappears from peripheral blood T cells. T4 antigen appears to recognize the inducer/helper population and T5 antigen the suppressor/cytotoxic population of T lymphocytes. T4 is present on approximately 60% of peripheral blood T lymphocytes and T5 on 20 to 30% of peripheral T lymphocytes. The T4+ cells provide inducer function in T–T, T–B, and T–macrophage interactions. T4+ cells alone are required to induce B cell differentiation into immunoglobulin-containing plasma cells. T cell helper factor that initiates B cell differentiation to immunoglobulin-synthesizing plasma cells is produced by the T4+ subset alone. The T5+ subset contains a population of cells with suppressor functions, both for T cell proliferation (T–T suppression) and B cell differentiation to immunoglobulin-synthesizing plasma cells (T–B suppression). Virtually 100% of peripheral blood T cells possess the antigen designated as T1 whereas only 10% of thymocytes possess this antigen. Furthermore, the latter thymocytes appear to be the functional thymocytes that can respond by proliferation in mixed leukocyte culture. Analysis of various antigens and consequently these subpopulations is done either by indirect immunofluorescence using a fluorescence-activated cell sorter, cytofluorograph, or complement-dependent cytotoxicity assay.

A number of investigators have developed monoclonal antibodies that define the total T cell population (Pan T) and permit definition of functionally distinct subpopulations of T lymphocytes. For example, Evans, now working in our laboratory, has developed antisera reactive with most thymocytes and almost all if not all peripheral blood T lymphocytes. He has designated this antigen as anti-Leu 1. Interestingly, this antiserum also recognized an antigen present on the malignant B lymphocytes in 11 of 14 patients with chronic lymphocytic leukemia. The Leu 1 antigen is, however, not present on normal B lymphocytes. This plus a molecular size and migration characteristic as a doublet in SDS–polyacrylamide gel provoked the speculation that this antigen might be the equivalent of the G IX determinant on GP 70 in the mouse. The latter is a debatable point and according to some data obtained in collaboration with Hertzenberg and associates the antigen may, indeed, be slightly smaller and may actually represent the human equivalent of Lyt 1. From recent fluorescence analysis with fluorescence-activated cell sorter and other techniques Lyt 1 has been found to be present on all T lymphocytes. Evans has also been studying four separate monoclonal antibodies which recognize two separate peptides present on the surface membranes of two major distinct subpopulations of human T lymphocytes. These antibodies are designated as anti-Leu 2a and anti-Leu 2b. These antisera recognize two different epitopes on a single peptide that distinguishes the suppressor/cytotoxic subset of human T cells. Indeed, these antisera recognize the same subpopulation of T lymphocytes that is recognized by the anti-TH2 rabbit antiserum originally described by Evans *et al.* (1978). Another subpopulation that contains cells capable of exerting helper functions in immunoglobulin synthesis and that is TH2 negative is recognized by two antisera designated anti-Leu 3a and anti-Leu 3b. Like the monoclonal antibodies described by Schlossman and his colleagues, those designated Leu 1, Leu 2a, Leu 3b, Leu 3a, and Leu 3b are being made commercially available.

Similar antisera capable of distinguishing functionally distinct subpopulations of human T lymphocytes have been prepared by Levy *et al.* (1979) of Stanford and Hansan *et al.* (1980) at the University of Washington in Seattle among others.

The molecular nature of the gene products responsible for the membrane antigenicity recognizable with these monoclonal antibodies is rapidly being defined. It is clear that these molecules will have important functional significance. For example, in work by Evans *et al.* (1978) in our laboratories already the anti-Leu 2a and to a lesser extent the anti-Leu 2b have been shown in the absence of added complement to be able to interfere with T cell-mediated cytotoxicity in the cell-mediated lympholysis assay.

C. Clinical Application of Monoclonal Antibodies

Monoclonal antibodies have potential application in diagnosis, classification, and therapy of certain lymphoproliferative and immunodeficiency disorders. One of the uses of multiple anti-T cell monoclonal antibodies has been in defining and classifying acute lymphoblastic leukemia (ALL) according to the stage of differentiation. Using these types of reagents it has been possible to correlate different types of ALL of T cell lineage with survival. Leukemic blasts from patients with Sezary syndrome bear the T4 antigen that defines the population of T cells in normals that contain inducer/helper activity.

In certain patients with primary immunodeficiency and in patients who have developed graft-versus-host disease following bone marrow transplantation, abnormalities of regulatory T cells have been described.

Monoclonal antibodies to viral antigens have also been produced. These reagents will serve with ever increasing frequency and effectiveness as ideal reference typing reagents. Because of the lack of limitation on production of an identical product, scientists throughout the world will be able to use virtually identical immunologic reagents; of even greater potential is the possibility of using monoclonal antibodies in therapy of parasitic disease, therapy and prevention of graft-versus-host disease, and even treatment of leukemias, lymphomas, and perhaps other cancers. Already in experimental systems it has been possible to prevent graft-versus-host reaction by eliminating unwarranted T cells which have already come under thymic influence and thus bear the Thy-1 antigen from bone marrow preparations prior to transplant and to treat leukemia of mice successfully using monoclonal antibodies. Ideal for therapeutic use in man will be to extend the hybridoma development to human myeloma so that antibody produced can be of human origin. Such antibodies may also be of immense value in the treatment of primary immunodeficiency diseases.

Recently Brouet and Seligmann have discovered that patients with Wiskott–Aldrich syndrome very frequently produce an antiserum that distinguishes a subpopulation of B lymphocytes. This subpopulation comprises 30–60% of lymphocytes in normal healthy adults, 60–90% in patients with the Wiskott–Aldrich syndrome, and only 3–20% in obligate carriers of the Wiskott–Aldrich syndrome. There is no question whatever that developmental stages of B lymphocytes can be defined with monoclonal antisera prepared by hybridoma technology in exactly the same way as has been done for T lymphocytes. This approach too will prove useful in better defining and perhaps ultimately treating leukemias, lymphomas, and immunodeficiencies involving malignancies and disturbances of B cell line lineages, e.g., autoimmunities.

XII. Relationship between Tγ Cells and Monocytes

Recently it has been shown that Tγ cells do not react with OK T5 antibody that defines suppressor/cytotoxic cells. By contrast subpopulations of Tγ cells have been found to react with monoclonal antibody that is said to define monocytes. Based on these observations, Reinherz et al. (1980) concluded that Tγ cells are not lymphocytes, but rather cells of monocyte lineage. They are not T cells at all. A number of objections can be raised against this interpretation. In the initial studies when monoclonal antibodies against T cells and T cell subsets were tested for their specificity and functions, purified T cells were obtained by rosetting with SRBC that were not treated with either neuraminidase or AET. Therefore, low-affinity E rosette-forming T cells would be left in the non-T cell fraction. Furthermore, it is known that among the low-affinity E rosette-forming T cells are Tγ cells. This could account for the unreactivity of Tγ cells with antibodies prepared against T cells. Similarly, the specificity of monoclonal antibody that defines monocyte was tested for reactivity with T cells that again had not been prepared by rosetting with neuraminidase-treated SRBC. Therefore the majority of Tγ cells would have been left in non-T cell fractions and not tested for the reactivity with antiserum. However, when analysis on Tγ cells was performed, T cells were purified by rosetting with neuraminidase-treated SRBC. Table II also lists the many differences between monocytes and Tγ cells which seem to indicate strongly that a large pro-

TABLE II
DIFFERENCES BETWEEN Tγ CELLS AND MONOCYTES

	Tγ cells	Monocytes
1. Rosettes with SRBC	+	−
2. Ingestion of latex particles	−	+
3. Nonspecific esterase	−	+
4. Locomotion toward chemoattractants	−	+
5. Proliferation to		
PHA	+	−
Con A	+	−
Staph protein A	+	−
6. Produce antigen-specific suppressor factor	+	−
7. Produce immune interferon (to PHA)	+	−
8. Modulation of Fc receptor by insoluble immune complexes	+	−
9. May develop upon exposure of peripheral blood T cells or the bone marrow to thymic hormone	+	−
10. Reactive with antibody against IgG Fc receptors from T cells	+	−
11. Can be grown as clonal cultures with T cell growth factor	+	−
12. Natural cytotoxicity in 2–4 hour assay	+	−

portion of Tγ cells are elements of T cell lineage. One might also suggest that Tγ cells are not mature monocytes, but rather promonocytes. However, this does not appear to be the case, because monoclonal antibodies that define the mature monocytes do not appear to react with promonocytes. It is important that these discrepancies be resolved. This could be done by using monoclonal antibodies with pan-T specificity, monoclonal antibodies against T cell subsets, and monoclonal antibody prepared against Tγ cells. From our own studies about 40–80% of Tγ cells appear to react with monoclonal antibody that defines cytotoxic/suppressor cell population of man. This is approximately the percentage of Tγ cells that have histamine receptors and exert suppressor activity. It is the other 50% of Tγ cells that mediate natural killing and antibody-dependent cytotoxicity. They lack receptors for histamine.

XIII. Distinction of Lymphocytes from Monocytes

The preponderant method of lymphocyte isolation in common use utilizes differences in cell density as a primary discrimination from other blood cells. The low-density fraction in these preparations contains both lymphocytes and monocytes. This mononuclear fraction contains 20 to 30% monocytes in normal individuals, but in chronic inflammatory diseases and lymphopenic states monocytes can greatly outnumber lymphocytes in this fraction. The particular problem posed by the monocyte is challenging because certain of the surface components of the monocyte are shared with the lymphocyte. These include complement receptors, Fc receptors, and Ia molecules. Furthermore, the presence of Fc receptors confers on the cells the ability to yield false-positive reactions by binding to the Fc portions of serum IgG or to antibodies used as reagents. Thus these cell can appear to possess surface Ig-like B cells. It is, however, possible, with care, to distinguish such monocytes from lymphocytes.

Depletion of monocytes may be accomplished by taking advantage of their adherence to plastic flask surfaces or to Sephadex G-10 beads. Furthermore, they can be distinguished or separated by their phagocytic property. For example, permitting them to ingest iron compounds or crystalline substances permits their removal by centrifugation or magnetic manipulation. One must, however, realize that B cells may also adhere to plastic surfaces, and thus some of these may be removed from the preparations being analyzed. Therefore, great caution must be exercised and it is necessary to ascertain just how a depletion procedure influences the lymphocyte populations.

The second approach is one of identification of the monocyte without any attempt at depletion. To a certain extent, this can be accomplished with phase microscopy utilizing as criteria the following characteristic morphological features: (1) the ruffled cytoplasmic membrane; (2) the larger more granular cytoplasm; and (3) the characteristic nuclear morphology of the mature monocyte. Supravital nuclear stains, such as toluidine blue or acridine orange, will also assist in making the distinction. When the cells are exposed to latex particles or bacteria, the phagocytic function permits recognition of the monocyte. All of these methods have potential for error since immature monocytes present in abundance in certain disease states are less distinctive in morphology and may phagocytize poorly. Furthermore, some adherent lymphocytes may bind the indicator particles on their surface membranes and, without special studies, it is difficult to distinguish phagocytosis from binding. Thus, a third alternative is to use biochemical properties of the monocyte as identifying markers. These include histochemical staining for nonspecific esterase or peroxidase.

Each of these approaches is effective to some degree under particular circumstances, but none is 100% effective in all situations. Thus, an awareness of the intriguing biology of the monocyte is essential for effective analysis of lymphocyte populations.

XIV. The Third-Cell Population or Unclassified Lymphoid Cells

One central question is whether the primary lymphocyte populations are those of the B cell and the T cell or whether the "third" or null cell population is a true additional population with a distinct significance. From the above review and elsewhere in this volume, it is evident that under certain conditions of assay approximately 5% of lymphocytes will be found to lack surface markers. But when additional assays are utilized or when the cell membranes are perturbed as with neuraminidase, the majority of these cells appear to enter either the B or T cell category. This finding suggests the interpretation that the appearance of "null cells" could be a common end state of particular differentiation pathways within both the T and the B lineage and might include such diverse entities as plasma cells and cells capable of mediating antibody-dependent cytotoxicity. A provisional conclusion is that the "third" population appears to be only an operationally useful classification and that major doubts exist regarding its existence as a completely independent and functionally separate lymphocyte lineage. A better interpretation seems to be that this population comprises many small subpopulations of cells basically distinct from one another and related to their lineages of the hematopoietic and lymphoid systems.

XV. Summary

Study of subpopulations of lymphocytes in man is now a highly developed field. Surface markers including receptors for complement components, receptors for several different immunoglobulins, differentiation antigens recognized by heteroantisera and monoclonal antibodies prepared by the hybridoma technologies as well as receptors for surface components of certain red blood cell antigens, and enzymes and lectins from a variety of sources have all been used to recognize and define lymphocyte subpopulations. The understanding of primary and secondary immunodeficiencies, the definition and analysis of lymphoreticular malignancies, the investigation of autoimmunities, and the understanding of the influences of persisting infections and modern chemotherapy and consequences of malignant diseases require the application of these techniques. Although apparently complex at this juncture, one can be assured that the future will bring progressive simplification as we learn to study and work with the networks of cells that stand as bulwarks of our bodily defense.

References

Evans, R. L., Lazarus, H., Penta, A. C., and Schlossman, S. F. (1978). Two functionally distinct subpopulations of human T cells that collaborate in the generation of cytotoxic cells responsible for cell-mediated lympholysis. *J. Immunol.* **120,** 1423–1428.

Good, R. A., and Finstad, J. (1980). Immunodeficiencies 1980. *Proc. Int. Conf. Immunodeficiency 3rd*, in press.

Gupta, S., and Good, R. A. (1979). Human T lymphocytes as defined by Fc receptors. *Thymus* **1,** 135–149.

Gupta, S., and Good, R. A. (1980). Markers of human lymphocyte subpopulations in primary immunodeficiency and lymphoproliferative disorders. *Seminars Hematol.* **17,** 1–29.

Gupta, S., Fernandes, G., Rocklin, R., and Good, R. A. (1980). Histamine receptors on human T cell subsets. *In* "New Trends in Human Immunology and Cancer Immunotherapy" (B. Serrou and C. Rosenfeld, eds.). Dion Editeur, Paris, in press.

Hansen, J. A., Martin, P. J., and Nowinski, R. C. (1980). Monoclonal antibodies identifying a novel T cell antigen and Ia antigen of human lymphocytes. *Immunogenetics* **10**, 247–260.

Ko, H. S., Fu, S. M., Winchester, R. J., Yu, D. T. Y., and Kunkel, H. G. (1979). Ia determinants on stimulated human T cells. *J. Exp. Med.* **150**, 246.

Levy, R., Dilley, J., Fix, R. I., and Warnke, R. (1979). Human thymus leukemia antigen defined by hybridoma monoclonal antibodies. *Proc. Natl. Acad. Sci. U.S.A.* **76**, 6552–6556.

Moretta, L., Ferrarini, M., and Cooper, M. D. (1978). Characterization of human T cell subpopulations as defined by specific receptors for immunoglobulins. *Contemp. Topics Immunobiol.* **8**, 19–53.

Reinherz, E. L., and Schlossman, S. F. (1980). The differentiation and function of human T lymphocytes. *Cell* **19**, 821–827.

Reinherz, E. L., Moretta, L., Roper, M., Breard, J. M., Mingari, M. C., Cooper, M. D., and Schlossman, S. F. (1980). Human T lymphocyte subpopulations defined by Fc receptors and monoclonal antibodies. A comparison. *J. Exp. Med.* **151**, 969–974.

Ross, G. D. (1979). Identification of human lymphocyte subpopulations by surface marker analysis. *Blood* **53**, 799–811.

Sjoberg, O. (1980). Presence of receptors for IgD on human T and non-T lymphocytes. *Scand. J. Immunol.* **11**, 377–382.

Wang, C. Y., Good, R. A., Ammirati, P., Dymbort, G., and Evans, R. L. (1980). Identification of a P69,71 complex expressed on human T cells sharing determinants with B type chronic lymphocytic leukemia. *J. Exp. Med.* **151**, 1539–1544.

Winchester, R. J., and Ross, G. (1976). Methods for enumerating lymphocyte subpopulations. *In* "Manual of Clinical Immunology" (N. R. Rose and H. Freedman, eds.), p. 64. American Society of Microbiology, Washington, D.C.

Winchester, R. J., Fu, S. M., Hoffman, T., and Kunkel, H. G. (1975). IgG on lymphocyte surfaces; technical problems and the significance of a third cell population. *J. Immunol.* **114**, 1210–1212.

Yodoi, J., and Ishizaka, K. (1979). Lymphocytes bearing Fc receptors for IgE. I. Presence of human and rat T lymphocytes with Fc receptors. *J. Immunol.* **122**, 2577–2583.

Lymphocyte Membrane Complement Receptors

GORDON D. ROSS[1]

Division of Rheumatology and Immunology,
University of North Carolina Medical School, Chapel Hill, North Carolina

I. Introduction	33
II. Methods for Detection of C Receptors	37
A. Rosette Assays	37
B. Fluorescence Assays	38
C. Specificity Controls	39
III. Expression of C Receptors and Other Surface Markers on Normal and Leukemic Human Lymphocytes	40
A. Surface Markers of Complement Receptor Lymphocyte (CRL) from Normal Blood	40
B. Expression of C Receptors on Blood Lymphocytes from Patients with Chronic Lymphatic Leukemia (CLL)	41
C. Expression of C Receptors on Blood Lymphocytes from Patients with Macroglobulinemia	42
D. CRL in the Tonsils, Spleen, and Thoracic Duct	42
IV. Interpretation and Significance	42
References	45

I. Introduction

Membrane receptors for serum complement (C) proteins are present on several different cell types including lymphocytes, neutrophils, eo-

---

[1] Established Investigator of the American Heart Association, and supported by a research grant from the National Cancer Institute (CA-25613).

sinophils, monocyte–macrophages, kidney glomerular cells, primate erythrocytes, and nonprimate platelets. The structure and specificity of the C receptors on these different cell types is very similar, if not identical. C receptors bind either fluid-phase C or C fixed onto antigen–antibody complexes (immune complexes). Because of their ability to bind to the C on immune complexes, C receptors cause immune complexes to become firmly attached to lymphocytes and in this way may possibly enhance detection of antigens by lymphocytes. C receptors thus function similarly to lymphocyte receptors for the antibody contained in immune complexes (Fc receptors, or FcR). C receptors, though, have a much higher binding energy than do Fc receptors, so that in a competitive situation antibody and C-coated antigens are bound to C receptors rather than to Fc receptors.

Studies of the role of the complement system in the immune response have demonstrated an important function for the third component, C3. Animals depleted of circulating C3 by treatment with cobra venom factor have a reduced or absent humoral response to thymus-dependent antigens (Pepys, 1974). Since this pathway of bone marrow-derived lymphocyte (B cell) activation by antigen requires both thymus-derived lymphocytes (T cells) and macrophages, it is unclear which cell type interacts with C3 and in what way. Since it has been shown that antigen trapping in lymph nodes and spleen is greatly reduced in C3-depleted animals, it has been suggested that the role of C3 is merely to crosslink antigen complexes to C receptors of B cells. However, complete inhibition of T cell-dependent responses has also been reported in lymphocyte tissue culture systems utilizing C3-deficient media, indicating that the role of C3 may go beyond antigen trapping in lymphoid follicles and may be involved in the process of lymphocyte activation (Lewis *et al.*, 1977). The exact role of C and of C receptors in the immune response to antigens remains unknown. The function of granulocyte and macrophage C receptors is more readily demonstrated than that of lymphocytes. C receptors on the membranes of these phagocytic cells greatly enhance their ability to ingest bacteria and yeast. In plasma, microbial organisms quickly become "opsonized" with a coating of C that causes them to stick to phagocyte C receptors. Once they are firmly attached to leukocyte membranes, the microbes are rapidly ingested and destroyed. Among lymphocytes there is a small population of non-B non-T cells that uses their C receptors in a similar manner. Killer cells (or K cells) that kill antibody and C-coated tumor cells have

C receptors that enhance this cytotoxic activity by binding the killer cells firmly to the C-coated tumor cells (Perlman et al., 1975).

Lymphocytes have been shown to bear two different types of C receptors, known as CR_1 and CR_2; CR_1 is known also as the C3b or immune adherence receptor; CR_2, as the C3d receptor. These two types of C receptors have different specificities, are structurally distinct, and are located on separate molecules within the lymphocyte membrane (Ross and Polley, 1975). Treatment of lymphocytes with various proteolytic enzymes abolishes C receptor activity, indicating that proteins make up an essential part of the C receptor structure. Three different C components bind to lymphocyte C receptors: C3, C4, and C5. These three proteins share a common structure that allows binding to CR_1 type receptors. In addition, C3 contains a second receptor binding site that is not found in either C4 or C5 and that binds C3 to CR_2 type receptors. Native plasma C3, C4, and C5 bind weakly to CR_1 and are readily displaced by the multivalent presentation of the activated "b" form of these C proteins, which is concentrated on the surface of immune complexes. By contrast, the CR_2 binding site in the C3 molecule is not exposed in native C3 and is revealed only subsequent to C3 activation and interaction with the modulating protein known as β1H.

Figure 1 is a schematic diagram of the specificity of lymphocyte C receptors. Activated C3, known as C3b, is shown at the top of the

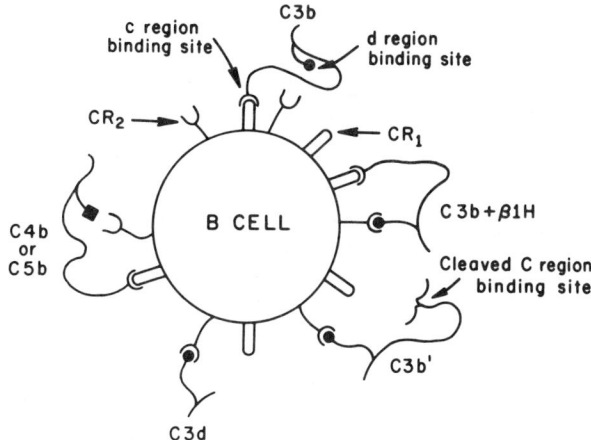

Fig. 1. Specificity of lymphocyte complement receptors.

figure. The site for CR_1 attachment is located in the "c" region of the C3b molecule, whereas the site for CR_2 attachment remains unexposed in the "d" region of C3b. Following interaction of C3b with the normal plasma protein β1H, the conformation of C3b is changed so as to expose the d region binding site for CR_2. This conformational change in C3b also renders the c region of C3b susceptible to cleavage by the plasma enzyme C3b inactivator. Cleavage of C3b by C3b inactivator destroys the c region binding site for CR_1, forming what is known as C3b' or C3bi. In plasma, C3b molecules are acted upon by both β1H and C3b inactivator, so that in a period of several minutes all of the C3b is converted to C3b'. This C3b' binds only to cells bearing CR_2 and no longer binds to cells bearing only CR_1. Additional serum proteases, such as plasmin, trypsin, elastase, or thrombin, then further degrade C3b' to the small C3d fragment. The C3d fragment, containing the fully active CR_2 binding site, remains firmly bound to immune complexes, whereas the larger C3c fragment is released from complexes into the fluid phase. C4b and C5b resemble C3b in that they have a site only for CR_1 attachment. However, degradation of C4b and C5b by plasma proteases destroys the CR_1 binding site without exposing any hidden binding sites for CR_2. *In vivo,* the most important function of C and C receptors is the clearance and destruction of microbial organisms. Since the mature neutrophils and macrophages that perform this function predominantly contain only CR_1 and lack CR_2, it has been proposed that C3b, either alone or in combination with β1H, is probably the most important C fragment in C receptor-mediated reactions. This is because quantitatively there is far more C3 in plasma than any other C component and because C3b can be generated by either the classical or alternative pathways of C activation. Under some circumstances though, it is also theoretically possible that either C4b or C5b could substitute for C3b. Indeed, phagocytic abnormalities have been reported in both mice and humans that are genetically deficient in C5.

In most cases, it is likely that C receptors react with C3 fragments bound to immune complexes rather than with single fluid phase C fragments. The multivalent presentation of C3 fragments on a complex has a much greater affinity for CRL than do individual fluid phase fragments, because many receptors are attached simultaneously. Such C3-coated complexes can form in two different ways. First, antigen–antibody complexes (immune complexes) activate the classical pathway of C activation beginning at C1 and ending at C9. Second, in the absence of specific antibody, the cell wall components of many strains of bacteria and yeast trigger the alternative pathway of C activation that begins with C3 and then terminates with C9. In either case, complexes containing C3b are generated that may then subsequently be bound to C receptors. This complex-bound C3b rapidly reacts with plasma β1H, generating the CR_2-reactive site in addition to the CR_1-reactive site. Cleavage of the CR_1-reactive site by C3b inactivator proceeds at a much slower rate, particularly on bacteria and yeast cell surfaces (Fearon and Austen, 1977), assuring that the CR_1 site remains active long enough to bind the complex to CR_1-bearing cells.

In addition to being found on B lymphocytes, CR_1 type receptors are also expressed on variable proportions of neutrophils, eosinophils, monocytes, and macrophages. On the other hand, these phagocytic cells lack CR_2 and express instead a third type of C receptor (CR_3) that binds only C3b', and not C3b or C3d. Erythrocytes differ from these other cell types in that they contain only CR_1.

II. Methods for Detection of C Receptors

Several different types of assay systems have been developed to detect C receptors. Generally, it has been found that C-coated particles that present multiple active sites for attachment to cells are better for detection of C receptors than the soluble individual C fragments.

A. Rosette Assays

Particles coated with C bind to complement receptor lymphocytes (CRL), forming a rosette around the lymphocyte that is easily visualized by phase-contrast microscopy. The type of C fragment that is present on the particles determines which type of C receptor is detected by the assay. If whole serum is used as a C source, the particles will usually contain predominantly C3b' or C3d and bind only to cells expressing CR_2. However, in some instances, particles generated with serum may also contain small but significant amounts of C3b-β1H, C4b, and C5b, so that the particles detect both CR_1 and CR_2 with nearly equal efficiency. For this reason, specialized techniques have been developed to control the process of C fixation onto the particles so that the particles contain only one reactive type of C fragment and thus specifically detect either CR_1 or CR_2.

Most commonly, erythrocyte–antibody–complement (EAC) complexes are prepared with either mouse, guinea pig, or human C. If serum from mice that are genetically deficient in C5 is used as a source of C, then the erythrocyte–antibody (EA) complexes may be treated with a high concentration of serum without causing C-mediated hemolysis. After prolonged treatment with the serum, the erythrocyte-bound C3b is eventually converted completely to C3b' and C3d, generating EAC complexes that specifically bind to lymphocyte CR_2. Preparation of EAC complexes that react specifically with CR_1 is more difficult. Ideally, the individual purified C components are added sequentially to the EA complexes until the stable EAC1 4b or EAC1 423b intermediate complex is formed. This, however, requires a large amount of the highly purified C proteins that are not available commercially. In the past, only laboratories specializing in C biochemistry could specifically assay lymphocyte CR_1. Recently though, a simpler short-cut procedure has been developed to prepare either EAC1 4b or EAC1 423b from serum, thus eliminating the need for purified C components (Ross and Polley, 1976).

In addition to sheep erythrocytes, the erythrocytes from other species have also been used to prepare EAC. Non-sheep E have been used primarily because it was found that sheep E bound to T cells lacking C receptors under certain conditions. However, the use of sodium azide in the assay media completely inhibits sheep E rosettes with T cells, since formation of T cell rosettes apparently requires an active oxidation metabolism, making the use of non-sheep E unnecessary. Also, bacteria and yeast (zymosan) have been used to form C-coated particles in combination with either specific antibody or direct activation of C by the alternative pathway. Use of alternative pathway-derived C, however, usually requires the use of whole serum as a source of C, and thus the same specificity problems are encountered as with the preparation of EAC with whole serum (Schreiber *et al.*, 1978).

B. Fluorescence Assays

Two basic types of fluorescence assays have been used to detect C receptors. In the first method, C-coated particles similar to those used for rosette assays are conjugated to either fluorescein or rhodamine. Frequently, heat-killed, C-coated bacteria are used, and these bind to CRL, forming a bright fluorescent rosette that is easily visualized by fluorescence microscopy. These small C-coated bacteria particles are advantageous to erythrocytes in that they may be stored frozen until use without loss of activity and are easily visualized in assays for C receptor cells in tissue sections. However, preparation of C-coated bacteria with whole serum can frequently lead to problems because of high-titer antibacterial IgG antibodies in serum that are difficult to absorb completely. If such antibodies coat the bacteria in addition to C, then the bacteria complexes may bind to Fc receptors on cells lacking C receptors and thus give false positive results.

The other type of fluorescence assay for C receptors utilizes fluorescein- or rhodamine-conjugated C3 fragments. Because of their single point of attachment, these fragments have a much lower affinity for CRL than do multivalent complexes heavily coated with C. The sensitivity of this assay can thus be greatly enhanced by aggregating the C3 fragments in some way to provide a higher affinity multipoint attachment to cells. One method for aggregating the fluorescent C3 fragments is to add a bivalent and fluorescence-labeled $F(ab')_2$ IgG anti-C3 to the cells subsequent to the uptake of the fluorescent C3 fragments. In this way, the weakly bound fluorescent C fragments are aggregated by the anti-C3 at the cell surface, stabilizing the attachment to C receptors. Monovalent fluorescence-labeled Fab IgG anti-C3, on the other hand, does not aggregate the fluorescent C3 fragments on the cell surface and, in fact, diminishes the binding of the C3 fragments by competing with C receptors for the binding sites in the C3 molecule.

C. Specificity Controls

Whatever type of C receptor assay is used, it is important that certain specificity controls be performed. Specificity for CR_1 is assured by a positive result with human erythrocytes, since these cells are known to contain CR_1 and totally lack CR_2. In addition, the same CR_1 assay should be negative with lymphocytes that contain only CR_2 and lack CR_1. The vast majority of cultured human lymphoblastoid cell lines have only CR_2, and thus are a valuable indicator for checking the specificity of the CR_1 assay system. The cell lines Daudi and Raji are now commonly being used in several laboratories and are recommended for this purpose. The CR_2 assay system must react in an opposite manner from the CR_1 assay, and so should be negative with human erythrocytes and positive with cultured lymphoblasts.

III. Expression of C Receptors and Other Surface Markers on Normal and Leukemic Human Lymphocytes

A. Surface Markers of Complement Receptor Lymphocyte (CRL) from Normal Blood

When C receptors were assayed by rosette formation with EAC1 4b or EAC1-3b (CR_1 specific) and EAC1-3b' or EAC1-3d (CR_2 specific), 17.0% of normal peripheral blood lymphocytes were found to express CR_1 and 9.4% to express CR_2. The cells bearing CR_2 were a subpopulation of the cells bearing CR_1, so that 9.4% of lymphocytes contained both types of C receptors ($CR_1^+CR_2^+$) and 7.6% contained only CR_1 ($CR_1^+CR_2^-$) (Table 1). Experiments that simultaneously labeled two or three different types of surface markers demonstrated that virtually all of the $CR_1^+CR_2^+$ cells also bore surface immunoglobulins (Ig) and determinants of Ia (histocompatiblity antigens encoded by I region genes and predominantly expressed on B cells, rather than T cells), confirming that they were members of the B cell lineage. Among the 7.6% $CR_1^+CR_2^-$ cells, 4.4% expressed either surface Ig or surface Ia, whereas the remaining 3.2% $CR_1^+CR_2^-$ cells lacked both of these B cell markers. The majority of the $Ia^-CR_1^+CR_2^-$ cells (2.1% out of 3.2%) did not express the T cell marker of sheep E rosette formation, whereas the remaining 1.1% simultaneously expressed both E rosette formation and CR_1 but lacked both surface Ig and Ia. Thus, it is possible

TABLE I
EXPRESSION OF C RECEPTORS ON NORMAL AND MALIGNANT LYMPHOCYTES

Lymphocyte source[a]	C receptor types detected		
	$CR_1^+CR_2^+$ (%)	$CR_1^+CR_2^-$ (%)	$CR_1^-CR_2^+$ (%)
Normal blood (21)	9.4	7.6	<0.5
Tonsils (14)	51	3.2	12
Spleen (3)	26	8.1	2.4
TDL[b] (5)	14	8.0	1.0
Chronic lymphatic leukemic blood (22)	21	2.2	45
Macroglobulinemic blood (4)	5.9	27	<0.5

[a] The number of samples examined is given in parentheses.
[b] TDL, thoracic duct lymphocytes.

that 1.1% of blood lymphocytes may be T cells that express CR_1. Receptors for the Fc portion of IgG (Fc receptors) were assayed by fluorescence with soluble antigen–antibody complexes conjugated to fluorescein or rhodamine. Fc receptors were detected on essentially all CRL, and an average of 12% of normal blood lymphocytes expressed Fc receptors and lacked C receptors.

Table II summarizes the correlation of the expression of C receptors with the expression of other types of surface markers. The various combinations of markers observed on normal blood lymphocytes defined five different subsets of CRL. The first three subsets belong to the B cell lineage because of their content of either Ig or Ia. The fourth and fifth subsets lacked Ig and Ia and thus cannot be classified as B cells. Even though cells of the fifth subset formed rosettes with sheep E, a T cell marker, the vast majority of T cell lacked C receptors, making it uncertain that these particular CR_1-bearing cells are T cells (Ross *et al.*, 1978b).

B. Expression of C Receptors on Blood Lymphocytes from Patients with Chronic Lymphatic Leukemia (CLL)

The differences between CR_1 and CR_2 type receptors was first recognized during studies of lymphocytes from patients with CLL. Many CLL lymphocytes typically expressed CR_2 and lacked CR_1. On the average, the lymphocytes from these patients contained twofold more CR_2^+ cells than CR_1^+ cells (Table I), and in some patients, 80% of the lymphocytes were $CR_1^- CR_2^+$. Such $CR_1^- CR_2^+$ cells were rare in normal blood, but made up a significant proportion of tonsil lymphocytes

TABLE II
Surface Marker-Defined Subsets of Normal Blood Complement Receptor (CR) Lymphocytes

CR type	Surface markers	Proportion (%)	Probable lineage
CR_1, CR_2	Ia, FcR, Ig	9.4	B cell
CR_1	Ia, FcR, Ig	2.0	B cell
CR_1	Ia, FcR	2.4	B cell
CR_1	FcR	2.1	?
CR_1	FcR, E rosette	1.1	?

(Table I). CR_2-bearing leukemic lymphocytes frequently did not express surface Ig, whereas nearly all normal blood CR_2-bearing cells had both Ig and CR_1.

C. Expression of C Receptors on Blood Lymphocytes from Patients with Macroglobulinemia

Blood lymphocytes from patients with Waldenström's macroglobulinemia differed markedly from CLL lymphocytes in that CR_1^+ cells greatly predominated over CR_2^+ cells (Table I). This population of $CR_1^+CR_2^-$ cells resembled normal blood $CR_1^+CR_2^-$ cells in that the majority did not express surface Ig (Ross and Polley, 1975).

D. CRL in the Tonsils, Spleen, and Thoracic Duct

Lymphocytes from tonsils were quite different in surface marker profile from normal blood lymphocytes, and in several ways more closely resembled leukemic blood lymphocytes (Table I). Among tonsil CRL, for example, there were more CR_2-bearing cells than CR_1-bearing cells, and the majority of $CR_1^-CR_2^+$ cells also lacked surface Ig. By contrast, spleen CRL contained more CR_1^+ than CR_2^+ cells, and similar to normal blood lymphocytes, most of the $CR_1^+CR_2^-$ cells lacked surface Ig. Thoracic duct CRL were very similar to peripheral blood CRL, and the higher proportion of CRL observed reflects the fact that the samples were taken from patients undergoing experimental chronic drainage of thoracic duct lymph. This procedure is known to deplete T cells selectively and thus increase the relative proportion of B cells. Lymph samples taken at weekly intervals showed progressive increases in the proportion of CRL (B cells).

IV. Interpretation and Significance

The exact function of C and C receptors in the immune response is unclear. Complement, in particular C3, has been shown to be an essential component of the humoral response to those certain antigens that are primarily recognized by T cells (Pepys, 1974; Lewis et al., 1977). Since this type of reaction is known to involve at least three different cell types (T cells, B cells, macrophages), one might expect the C receptors of either B cells or macrophages to be important in the immune response. In this regard, it may be significant that macrophages normally synthesize C3 and store at least part of this C3 on their cell surface CR_1. In tissue spaces devoid of C3, macrophages would thus have their own supply of C3 ready for use. Previous studies have suggested two possible roles for C receptors in the immune response. First, T cell-activated macrophages may generate C3b, C3b', or C3d fragments that subsequently react with B cell C receptors, triggering B cell activation (Dukor et al., 1974; Hartmann and Bokisch, 1976). Second, it has been suggested that antigens may form immune complexes with small amounts of circulating IgM "natural antibody" and thereby acquire a coating of classical pathway-derived C3b. Such C3-bearing complexes would then be concentrated on macrophage surfaces by way of C receptors, and, thus positioned, the C3 might then subsequently cross-link B cells to the macrophage surface, greatly enhancing antigen presentation to the B cells. Evidence for the first hypothesis comes from in vitro experiments in which C3b-supplemented media were shown to activate lymphocytes (Hartmann and Bokisch, 1975) and C3-deficient media were shown not to support T cell-dependent antibody responses (Lewis et al., 1977). The second hypothesis was supported by the finding that antigen trapping in the spleen did not occur in animals previously depleted of C3. Additional types of tests will be required to elucidate the exact function of C receptors in the immune response.

The function of C receptors is better understood in the case of certain non-B non-T lymphocytes that kill antibody-coated target cells. Such lymphocytes, often referred to as "killer cells" or K cells, utilize C receptors to enhance their attachment to antibody and C-coated target cells. The actual cell-mediated killing though, is triggered by the interaction of K cell Fc receptors with the IgG antibody coating, and a C coating alone does not induce this type of cytotoxicity even though it firmly attaches the K cells to the target cells (Perlman et al., 1975).

Despite our lack of knowledge about the function of C receptors, studies of the distribution of C receptors on different lymphocyte types have indicated that C receptors are a valuable B cell marker and thus of benefit in defining the lineage of various lymphocyte subpopulations. In particular, C receptors are occasionally expressed on certain Ia-bearing B cells that lack easily detectable surface Ig (Ross et al., 1978a). Even though there is still some question as to whether some small numbers of non-B cells may also express C receptors, it is clear that most, if not all, normal T cells lack C receptors.

Even though the majority of CRL express both CR_1 and CR_2 simultaneously, it has been of considerable interest to determine why minor proportions of CRL express either one type of C receptor or the other. Evidence accumulated from studies of mouse B cell differentiation has indicated that C receptor expression correlates with the stage of B cell maturation (Hämmerling et al., 1976). Even though these particular studies did not attempt to distinguish CR_1 from CR_2 expression, there is other evidence for differentiation-linked sequential expression of C receptors obtained from the examination of non-lymphoid cell differentiation (Rabellino et al., 1978; Ross et al., 1978a). During the maturation of both human and mouse neutrophils, immature myeloid cells first acquire membrane CR_3 and then at a later stage of development express also CR_1. Similar studies of human B lymphocyte differentiation have been difficult because, unlike cells of the myeloid series, cells representing various stages of lymphoid cell maturation cannot be distinguished by easily recognizable morphological features. However, there is good suggestive evidence that the marker expression sequence of developing B lymphocytes may parallel that of the myeloid series. Immature appearing Ia-positive lymphoblasts from patients with acute lymphoblastic leukemia usually have no detectable C receptors, whereas more mature-appearing lymphocytes from patients with chronic lymphatic leukemia express only CR_2 and lack CR_1. Among normal B cells, such $CR_2^+CR_1^-$ cells are rare in peripheral blood and spleen (which would be expected to contain predominantly mature B cells), but make up a significant proportion of bone marrow and tonsil B cells. The majority of normal blood and spleen B cells express both CR_1 and CR_2 simultaneously, whereas the remaining B cells from these lymphoid sources express only CR_1 and lack CR_2. Thus, it is likely that immature B cells express either no C receptors or only CR_2, whereas mature B cells express both types of C receptors or only CR_1.

Not only is there probably a definite sequence for C receptor appearance, but it has also been shown in other more definitive studies that surface Ig, Ia, and Fc receptors appear in a definite sequence. This probably explains to some extent why normal lymphocytes are made up of such a variety of different surface marker-defined subsets (such as those of Table II). Particularly among the Ia-positive cells of the B cell lineage, it is likely that these subsets merely represent progressive stages in a common pathway of B cell differentiation, rather than functionally distinct B cell subtypes. More information is likely to come from experiments in which various marker-defined subsets are isolated and examined in tissue culture for both cell differentiation and functional activity.

References

Dukor, P., Schumann, G., Gisler, R. J., Dierich, M., Konig, W., Hadding, U., and Bitter-Suermann, D. (1974). Complement-dependent B-cell activation by cobra factor and other mitogens. *J. Exp. Med.* **139**, 337.

Fearon, D. T., and Austen, K. F. (1977). Activation of the alternative pathway due to the resistance of zymosan-bound amplification convertase to endogenous regulatory mechanisms. *Proc. Natl. Acad. Sci. U.S.A.* **74**, 1683.

Hämmerling, U., Chin, A. F., and Abbott, J. (1976). Ontogeny of murine B lymphocytes: Sequence of B-cell differentiation from surface-immunoglobulin-negative precursors to plasma cells. *Proc. Natl. Acad. Sci. U.S.A.* **73**, 2008.

Hartmann, K.-U., and Boksich, V. A. (1976). Stimulation of murine B lymphocytes by isolated C3b. *J. Immunol.* **116**, 1735.

Lewis, G. K, Ranken, R., and Goodman, J. W. (1977). Complement dependent and independent pathways of T cell–B cell cooperation. *J. Immunol.* **118**, 1744.

Pepys, M. B. (1974). Role of complement in induction of antibody production in vivo. Effect of cobra factor and other C3-reactive agents on thymus-dependent and thymus-independent antibody response. *J. Exp. Med.* **140**, 126.

Perlman, P., Perlmann, H., and Müller-Eberhard, H. J. (1975). Cytotoxic lymphocytic cells with complement receptors in human blood. Induction of cytolysis by IgG antibody but not by target cell-bound C3. *J. Exp. Med.* **141**, 287.

Rabellino, E. M., Ross, G. D., Trang, H. T. K., Williams, N., and Metcalf, D. (1978). Membrane receptors of mouse leukocytes. II. Sequential expression of membrane receptors and phagocytic capacity during leukocyte differentiation. *J. Exp. Med.* **147**, 434.

Ross, G. D., and Polley, M. J. (1975). Specificity of human lymphocytic complement receptors. *J. Exp. Med.* **141**, 1163.

Ross, G. D., and Polley, M. J. (1976). Assay for the two diffferent types of lymphocyte complement receptors. *Scand. J. Immunol. Suppl.* **5**, 99.

Ross, G. D., Jarowski, C. I., Rabellino, E. M., and Winchester, R. J. (1978a). Sequential appearance of Ia-like antigens and two different complement receptors during the maturation of human neutrophils. *J. Exp. Med.* **147**, 730.

Ross, G. D., Winchester, R. J., Rabellino, E. M., and Hoffman, T. (1978b). Surface markers of complement receptor lymphocytes. *J. Clin. Invest.* **62**, 1086.

Schreiber, R. D., Pangburn, M. K., Lesavre, P. H., and Müller-Eberhard, H. J. (1978). Initiation of the alternative pathway of complement: recognition of activators by bound C3b and assembly of the entire pathway from six isolated proteins. *Proc. Natl. Acad. Sci. U.S.A.* **75**, 3948.

Regulatory Human T-Cell Subpopulations Defined by Receptors for IgG or IgM

LORENZO MORETTA and MAX D. COOPER

Istituto di Microbiologia, University of Genoa, Genoa, Italy, and Cellular Immunobiology Unit of the Tumor Institute, Departments of Pediatrics and Microbiology, and The Comprehensive Cancer Center, University of Alabama in Birmingham, Birmingham, Alabama

I. Introduction	47
II. Enumeration and Isolation of T_M and T_G Cells	48
III. Morphology of T_M and T_G Cells	49
IV. Tissue Distribution of T_M and T_G Cells	50
V. Functional Analysis of T_M and T_G Cells	50
VI. Clinical Relevance of T_M and T_G Subpopulations	52
Selected Reading	53
Addendum	53

I. Introduction

Despite their rather uniform appearance, thymus-derived (T) lymphocytes are by no means a homogeneous population. Evidence obtained over the last few years indicates great functional heterogeneity of T cells. They mediate a wide spectrum of immune responses, such as rejection of foreign grafts, delayed hypersensitivity, antiparasitic immunity, rejection of cells antigenically modified by malignant transformation or viral infection. In addition, T cells exert both helper and suppressor control of antibody responses, thus playing a central regulatory role for humoral immunity. In mice these various properties have been attributed to distinct classes and subclasses of T cells identified by different membrane markers. Thus, T cells bearing Ly1 alloantigens usually exert helper activity on the antibody response, respond to alloantigens in mixed lymphocyte cultures (MLC), and are primarily responsible for delayed hypersensitivity reactions. Ly2 and 3 alloantigens usually characterize suppressor and cytotoxic T cells. Another useful way to look at murine T lymphocyte subtypes was recently provided by detection of Fc receptors for IgG on a subpopulation of normal mouse T lymphocytes. This made it possible to correlate the various functions of T lymphocyte subpopulations with the presence or the absence of the receptors for the crystallizable portion (Fc) of IgG.

The possibility to enumerate functionally defined, T-cell subpopulations in humans is clearly needed to understand pathogenic mechanisms involved in various immunological disorders and eventually to exert precise therapeutic control over immune responses. Information about human T cell subsets has been relatively difficult to acquire owing to problems in antisera specific for surface alloantigens on T cells and other obvious constraints for human investigation.

One means of identifying human T cell subpopulations was provided by the observation that T lymphocytes from normal individuals have surface receptors for the Fc portion of IgG and the discovery of a new T cell receptor with high avidity for the terminal Fc end of IgM molecules. Both IgG and IgM receptors identify only a proportion of circulating T lymphocytes; one T cell apparently carries receptors for only one or the other immunoglobulin. Therefore receptors for IgG and IgM represent useful markers for two distinct subpopulations of T cells, which, for simplicity, have been called T_G (or $T\gamma$) and T_M (or $T\mu$).

II. Enumeration and Isolation of T_M and T_G Cells

Mononuclear cells (lymphocytes and monocytes) can be isolated from erythrocytes and granulocytes by centrifugation of Ficoll–Hypaque density gradients. Most of the monocytes adhere to plastic surfaces and can be removed by incubating mononuclear cell suspensions in plastic dishes. Human T cells can be recognized and isolated by their special capacity to bind sheep erythrocytes (E) spontaneously, i.e., to form E rosettes. This binding is stable at low temperatures. Lymphocytes bound to erythrocytes are "heavier" as compared with free lymphocytes; thus E-rosetting T cells can be isolated from nonrosetting ones on density gradient centrifugation. After disruption of rosettes by vigorous shaking, the sheep erythrocytes can be separated from the purified T cells on Ficoll–Hypaque gradients carried out at 37°C. This temperature will prevent the reassociation of sheep erythrocytes with the T lymphocytes. T cells with receptors for IgG or for IgM are then detected and enumerated by secondary rosette formation using bovine erythrocytes coated either with purified IgG or with IgM antibodies. This is a relatively simple technique. In addition, cells forming rosettes with either IgG- or IgM-coated erythrocytes can be isolated on Ficoll–Hypaque gradients. Adherent red cells in this case are removed by osmotic lysis.

III. Morphology of $T._M$ and $T._G$ Cells

Although all T cells share general morphological similarity, light and electron microscopic examination of purified $T._M$ and $T._G$ populations has revealed interesting morphological and histochemical differences. Thus $T._M$ cells exhibit the characteristics of typical small lymphocytes, with a thin rim of basophilic cytoplasm and dense accumulations of nuclear chromatin. In contrast, $T._G$ lymphocytes are slightly larger, have a more abundant and weakly basophilic cytoplasm, and contain azurophilic granules, which vary in size, number, and distribution. These granules do not contain the enzyme markers of lysosomes present in macrophages and granulocytes. The nuclear chromatin of $T._G$ cells is more homogeneously distributed as compared to $T._M$ cells. Examination by electron microscopy reveals that, in comparison with $T._M$ cells, the cytoplasm of $T._G$ cells is rich in mitochondria, rough endoplasmic reticulum, and Golgian cisternae. The azurophilic granules of $T._G$ cells are surrounded by a membrane unit and contain an electron-dense material. The biochemical nature of the vesicle-enclosed material, which may be rapidly released following surface binding of IgG immune complexes, has yet to be defined. A very practical marker for $T._M$ cells is provided by the presence of large cytoplasmic accumulations of nonspecific esterase activity, which can be easily discerned on an appropriately stained blood smear.

IV. Tissue Distribution of T_M and T_G Cells

T_M and/or T_G cells are present in significant but varying proportions in all lymphoid tissues, with the remarkable exception of the thymus. Thus T_M cells are present in large proportions in peripheral blood, tonsils, and lymph nodes; T_G cells outnumber T_M cells in the spleen, but are detectable in much lower proportions in the other lymphoid organs and may be completely absent in normal unstimulated lymph nodes. An interesting observation is the detection of elevated proportions of T_G cells in the blood of newborns.

Since thymocytes are immature T cells, the paucity of T_M and T_G cells in the thymus suggests that the receptors for IgG or IgM are expressed by T cells at later stages in their development. Variations in the expression of other membrane components during the maturational process of T lymphocytes are known to occur in the mouse. T cell precursors acquire most of the T cell-specific antigens, such as GIX, Thy-1, TL, and Ly, within the mouse thymus. "Mature" T lymphocytes present in peripheral lymphoid organs of the mouse lack GIX and TL antigens and express a smaller amount of Thy-1 antigen. In addition, subsets of mouse T cells selectively lose Ly surface alloantigens. Thus, in the periphery, cells carrying all the Ly alloantigens present on thymocytes (Ly1, 2, and 3) coexist with cells that have lost either Ly1 or Ly2 and 3 alloantigens.

V. Functional Analysis of T_M and T_G Cells

Responses to mitogens, such as phytohemagglutinin (PHA) or concanavalin A (Con A), and to cells bearing different histocompatibility antigens are normally used as *in vitro* measures of the functional capabilities of T cells. T_M and T_G subpopulations of cells have therefore been analyzed for their responsiveness to these T cell mitogens and to major histocompatibility alloantigens. Whereas the responses to Con A are similar for all the T cell populations tested, significant differences can be detected in the response patterns of T_M and T_G cells to PHA and histocompatibility alloantigens. The normal immune response almost certainly involves regulatory interactions between T cells belonging to the different subpopulations.

The major functional difference so far detected between T_M and T_G

subpopulations concerns their regulatory control over antibody production by B cells. To show this we have used a convenient *in vitro* model system—the response of B cells to pokeweed mitogen (PWM). PWM induces polyclonal lymphocyte proliferation and maturation of B lymphocytes into antibody-secreting cells. After PWM stimulation a proportion of cells develop the morphological characteristics of plasmablasts and plasma cells. The cytoplasm of these cells contains large amounts of immunoglobulins that are easily detectable by immunofluorescent staining of fixed cytocentrifuge preparations and are secreted in the culture fluid in amounts measurable by radioimmunoassay. B cell maturation in this and other study systems is dependent upon the presence of T lymphocytes. Therefore the *in vitro* response of B lymphocytes to PWM offers a convenient model system for evaluating the mechanisms of immunoregulation exerted by T lymphocytes on B cell responses in humans.

In order to identify the T cell subpopulation(s) that induces B cells to differentiate and to make antibodies, B lymphocytes can be mixed with the various T cell populations and PWM. Help is assessed after 7 days in culture by measuring the numbers of cytoplasmic Ig-containing cells or the amount of secreted immunoglobulin. Using this system, only the T_M cells induce B cell maturation as well or better than unfractionated T lymphocytes. B cell differentiation is not observed in enriched B cell cultures supplemented with T_G lymphocytes. T cell populations depleted of T_M cells do not induce significant B cell maturation. Thus, T cells with helper activity are apparently restricted to the T_M cell population.

T_G cells, as $Ly2, 3^+$ lymphocytes in mice, have the property of suppressing antibody production. The mechanisms for the suppressor phenomenon has been studied by adding T_G lymphocytes to mixtures of helper T_M cells, B cells, and PWM. When added early, activated T_G cells can efficiently suppress B cell differentiation. The suppressor capacity is completely abrogated by γ-irradiation of T_G cells prior to culture. Suppressor capability is an exclusive property of the T_G cell subpopulation. T_M cells, macrophages, and B cells lack suppressor activity in this assay. T_G cell-suppressor activity is dependent upon cell interaction with both IgG immune complexes and PWM; after this double signal, T_G cells release soluble suppressor factors that prevent B cell differentiation by inhibiting T_M cell help. Thus the negative regulatory control that T_G cells exert on antibody responses by B cells occurs indirectly via a T suppressor–T helper interaction. The helper and suppressor capacities of T_M and T_G cells, respectively, has also been documented in antigen-specific assays *in vitro*.

VI. Clinical Relevance of T_M and T_G Subpopulations

It is reasonable to assume that T_M and T_G cells play important regulatory roles for antibody responses *in vivo*. Thus, both numerical and/or functional alterations in these T cell subpopulations could be expected in immunological disorders and may be involved in the pathogenesis of these diseases. Alterations of the proportions and/or of the functions of T_M and T_G are usually detectable in blood samples of patients with (*a*) congenital or acquired abnormalities of the thymus; (*b*) severe combined immunodeficiency; or (*c*) unexplained primary deficiency of cell-mediated immunity. Most of these patients have extremely low proportions of circulating helper T_M cells, often accompanied by increased proportions of T_G cells. Abnormally high numbers of T_G cells are found in patients affected by thymomas with immunodeficiency. Moreover, removal of T_G cells can completely abrogate suppressor activity elicited by unfractionated T lymphocytes from such patients.

Imbalances of T cell subpopulations have been infrequently detected in other immunodeficiency disorders, such as common variable hypogammaglobulinemia, X-linked agammaglobulinemia, and selective IgA deficiency. These observations are consistent with the idea that a variety of primary abnormalities may be responsible for antibody deficiencies in individuals with normal numbers of B lymphocytes. The defective B cell response could reflect functional defects of helper T cells, excessive activity of suppressor T cells, other aberrations in the cooperative interactions between T and B cells, or an inherent B cell defect.

In systemic lupus erythematosus (SLE) the excessive production of antibodies, many of which are directed against self-antigens, may be the consequence of defective suppressor T cell activity. SLE patients often show very reduced numbers of T_G lymphocytes, particularly when studied during active stages of the disease. This might be explained by the presence of cytotoxic antilymphocytic antibodies that specifically remove T_G cells. This possibility is made more reasonable by the demonstration of antibodies specific for suppressor T cells in patients with active juvenile rheumatoid arthritis. Another pertinent observation is that T_G cells lose their Fc receptors for an extended time period following interaction with IgG immune complexes. A similar phenomenon may occur *in vivo* in the course of diseases such as SLE, i.e., conditions in which high levels of circulating immune complexes exist. Since *in vitro* studies show that T_G cells suppress only after reaction with IgG immune complexes, then "modulation" of Fc receptors in SLE and other immune complex diseases could render T_G cells unable to receive an effective signal needed to regulate injurious immune responses.

Little research has been done with regard to expression of immunoglobulin (Ig) receptors on T cell leukemia and lymphomas. So far, receptors for IgM have been found on most acute lymphoblastic leukemias of the T cell type, but a few have expressed both IgM and IgG receptors, and some T cell leukemias apparently lack both types of receptors.

The pathogenesis of a variety of diseases and better therapeutic strategies are likely to become apparent as more is learned about these subpopulations of human T cells, and the nature and functional roles of their receptors for immunoglobulins, and other functional subsets of immunoregulatory T cells.

Selected Reading

Boyce, E. A., and Cantor, H. (1977). *Hospital Practice* 12, 81–88.
Grossi, C. E., Webb, S. R., Zicca, A., Lydyard, P. M., Moretta, L., Mingari, M. C., and Cooper, M. D. (1978). *J. Exp. Med.* 147, 1405–1417.
Gupta, S., and Good, R. A. (1977). *Clin. Exp. Immunol.* 30, 222.
Moretta, L., Mingari, M. C., Webb, S. R., Pearl, E. R., Lydyard, P. M., Grossi, C. E., Lawton, A. R., and Cooper, M. D. (1977a). *Eur. J. Immunol.* 7, 696–700.
Moretta, L., Webb, S. R., Grossi, C. E., Lydyard, P. M., and Cooper, M. D. (1977b). *J. Exp. Med.* 146, 184–199.

Addendum

Recent studies using monoclonal antibodies to differentiation antigens of mononuclear cells reveal two cell types in T_G preparations. Most (~75%) lack T cell antigens and share an antigen with macrophages; we speculate that these morphologically distinct cells are natural killer (NK) cells.

Mitogens

JOHN D. STOBO

Section of Rheumatology and Clinical Immunology, Moffitt Hospital,
University of California, San Francisco, California

I. Introduction	55
II. Fundamentals of Lectin-Induced Mitogenesis	57
III. Procedure for Determining *in Vitro* Lectin-Induced Activation of Lymphocytes	62
IV. Clinical Usefulness of Lectins	65
A. Influence of Soluble Serum Factors	67
B. Abnormalities at the Level of the Macrophages	69
C. Imbalances in Regulatory T Cells	69
General Reading References	72

I. Introduction

Several investigators working in the late 1800s and early 1900s demonstrated that substances isolated from plants had remarkable ability to agglutinate red blood cells from several animal species, including man. It soon became apparent that these phytohemagglutinins (*phyto* meaning isolated from plants) represented a series of proteins and glycoproteins that could interact with specific carbohydrate residues present in glycoproteins and glycolipids on the surface of many different cells. However, it was observed that diffferent cells within a species as well as the same type of cell (red blood cell, for example) from different species carried the carbohydrate ligands specific for some, but not other, phytohemagglutinins. Based on this specificity, the phytohemagglutinins were referred to as lectins (from the Latin *legere,* to pick or choose).

The usefulness of lectins in exploring lymphocyte biology and function was initiated by the observations of Peter C. Nowell (1960). While investigating agents suitable for chromosomal analysis of cells, Nowell discovered that small, quiescent resting lymphocytes could be stimulated to develop into lymphoblasts and divide (a process termed blastogenesis) by a phytohemagglutinin isolated from the red kidney bean. Thus, while lectins did not evolve for the convenience of cell biologists and immunologists (they probably perform an important function in the recognition process between plants and necessary nitrogen-fixing bacteria), they have served as invaluable probes for exploring lymphocyte biology.

In general, lectins are large (MW >60,000) molecules with multiple binding sites capable of interacting with specific carbohydrates present on lymphocyte cell surfaces. Thus, they fulfill two major criteria necessary for lymphocyte activation: they bind to lymphocyte surface; and their multivalent binding allows cross-linking of surface molecules providing membrane perturbation sufficient for activation. The usefulness of mitogens in studies of lymphocyte differentiation and function is based on two observations. First, metabolic and immunological events occurring during lectin-induced activation mimic, for the most part, those occurring during activation of lymphocytes by specific antigens. Second, in contrast to the relatively small frequency of lymphocytes (<1%) responsive to a single antigen, large portions (40–60%) of lymphocytes can be activated by lectins. In other words, while a given antigen activates only a single clone of specific immunocytes, lectins are polyclonal in that they activate many different clones of antigen-specific lymphocytes.

Over 100 different lectins isolated from a variety of plant and animal species have been studied. Although many of these are mitogenic, other actually inhibit lymphocyte blastogenesis. In this chapter, the usefulness of three common, mitogenic lectins—concanavalin A (Con A), phytohemagglutinin (PHA), and pokeweed mitogen (PWM)—in delineating human lymphocyte differentiation and function will be discussed.

II. Fundamentals of Lectin-Induced Mitogenesis

An understanding of the usefulness of lectins as probes for human lymphocyte biology requires a knowledge of immunocyte heterogeneity. Although this is more completely discussed in this volume by Winchester, a brief summary follows. Basically, three distinct populations of immunocompetent cells exist—T cells, B cells, and macrophages. T cells represent lymphocytes that have undergone a period of initial differentiation in the thymus and subsequently have passed to peripheral lymphoid tissue. T cells not only contain effector cells required to initiate cell-mediated reactions, but also contain distinct regulatory populations capable of "helping" (Th) or suppressing (Ts) several different immunological reactivities. In man, the total population of T cells is depicted by the presence of surface receptors for sheep red blood cells. In addition, Th bear a receptor specific for the Fc portion of IgM (Fcμ) and Ts display receptors for the Fc region of IgG (Fcγ).

In the fetus B lymphocytes undergo their initial differentiation in the liver, but in adults they differentiate within the bone marrow. Peripheralized B cells contain the precursors of antibody-secreting plasma cells and display easily detectable surface immunoglobulin determinants (IgM, IgD, or both IgM + IgD). B cells also contain Fc receptors and receptors capable of binding to certain components of activated complement.

While the exact ontogeny of macrophages is not well defined, they presumably derive from stem cells present in the bone marrow. Factors involved in the differentiation of stem cells → circulating monocytes → tissue macrophages are similarly not well delineated. In addition to their generalized function as phagocytes, macrophages serve to present antigens in a manner suitable for activation of T cells and B cells. While macrophages also bear Fc and complement receptors, their phagocytic properties and abundance of certain cytoplasmic enzymes serves to distinguish them from lymphocytes. Within this framework of lymphocyte heterogeneity, it is possible to examine events involved in the activation of lymphocytes by lectins (Fig. 1).

As previously indicated, polyclonal activation of lymphocytes by mitogens serves as a model for the activation of specific immunoreactive clones by antigen. Just as macrophages are crucially involved in

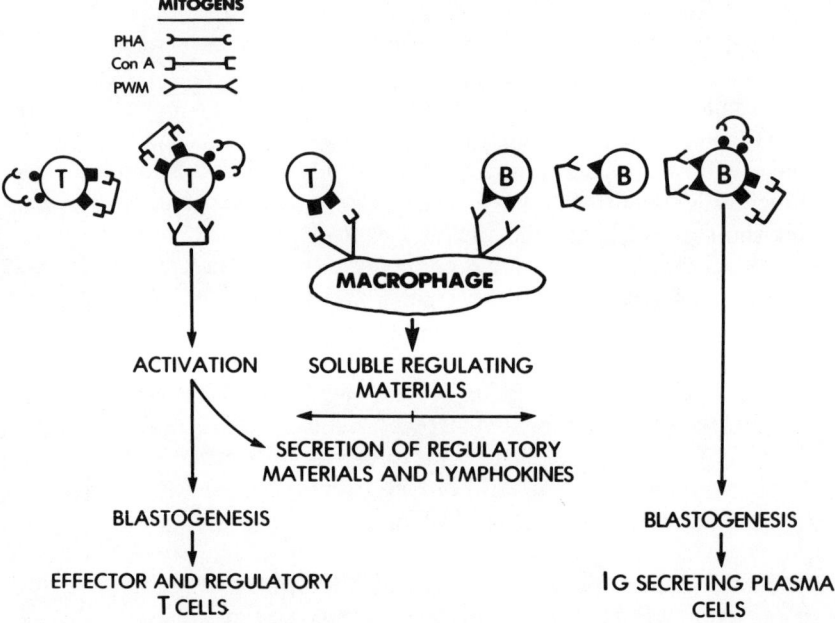

Fig. 1. Lectin-induced activation. This is a pictorial representation of lectin-induced activation of lymphocytes as outlined in the text. Among salient points are that (*a*) each lectin manifests specificity for distinct cell surface carbohydrate ligands; (*b*) phytohemagglutinin (PHA) and concanavalin A (Con A) activate predominantly T cells whereas pokeweed mitogen (PWM) activates T and B cells; (*c*) macrophages play a role in activation by "presenting" lectin and by secreting soluble materials that can amplify or suppress blastogenesis; (*d*) PHA- or Con A-induced secretion of immunoactive materials does not require blast transformation; (*e*) substantial B cell proliferation induced by PWM is regulated by T cells. Carbohydrate ligands: ●, *N*-acetyl-D-glucosamine; ■, mannopyranose; ▲ ?

the immune response to antigens, macrophages also play a key role in initial afferent events required for lectin-induced mitogenesis. This macrophage involvement is manifested in three ways. First, there exists a portion of T cells that cannot be directly activated by the simple binding of mitogens (PHA and Con A) to their surface. Instead, they are best activated by mitogen that is presented or initially processed by the macrophage. Second, a population of lymphocytes exists among which low levels of activation can be initiated by direct interactions between lectins and surface receptors. However, the subsequent blastogenesis of this population is markedly enhanced by soluble "facilitating" factors liberated by macrophages. Finally, macrophages can also liberate soluble materials (prostaglandins, for example) that are capable of suppressing lectin-induced blastogenesis. Thus, macrophages are involved in the initiation and subsequent regulation of lectin-induced mitogenesis.

It should be emphasized that the bulk of the work delineating the role of macrophages in mitogen-induced blastogenesis has been performed in murine systems utilizing PHA and Con A. However, an analogous situation most likely pertains to PHA-, Con A-, and PWM-induced blastogenesis in man.

Assuming that macrophages are required for initial activation and subsequent regulation of mitogenesis, a crucial question concerns the nature of the lymphocytes subjected to these regulatory influences. Phytohemagglutinin and Con A have been termed T cell mitogens in that 80–90% of the induced blast cells derive from T cells whereas the remainder are of B cell origin. In contrast, roughly 50% of PWM-induced blasts are of T cell and 50% are of B cell origin. A key point is that B cell activation by all three mitogens is T dependent. Soluble PHA, Con A, or PWM are unable to induce substantial proliferation among B cells in the absence of T cells. This B cell activation appears to require some initial interaction between the mitogens and T cells as *in vitro* B cell proliferation occurs 1–2 days after T cell activation.

Although T cell populations responsive to PHA are also responsive to Con A, and vice versa, certain T cells may demonstrate preferential reactivity to one or the other of these mitogens. Of most importance is that preferential reactivity may correlate with certain stages of differentiation or functional properties of a given T cell subpopulation. For example, while Con A can induce substantial blastogenesis among mouse thymocytes, these relatively immature T cells respond poorly to PHA. Peripheralized T cells that differ in their location and function also demonstrate differential PHA/Con A reactivities. The relative PHA/Con A reactivity for T cells in the peripheral blood, lymph nodes, and spleen is 1.5/1, 1/1, and 0.8/1, respectively. Moreover, helper T cells (Th) are included among those T cells manifesting the highest PHA/Con A ratio whereas suppressive (Ts) and cytotoxic T cells are included among those most responsive to Con A.

Based on these observations, it might appear that the differential reactivity of T cells to PHA and to Con A could serve as useful probes for maturational and functional T cell populations. Indeed, early studies designed to delineate functional T cell heterogeneity utilized this as a marker for T cell subpopulations. However, subsequent studies have shown that the mechanisms responsible for a T cell population manifesting maximal reactivity to either PHA or to Con A are complex and do not simply correlate with the relative number of PHA or Con A molecules capable of binding to the cell surface. Moreover, at least in man, it appears that Con A reactivity may be more sensitive to macrophage–T cell interactions than PHA reactivity. Thus, a preferentially lower response to Con A could reflect some abnormality at the level of the macrophage rather than an intrinsic capability of the T cell population. Other markers such as Fcμ or Fcγ receptors have proved to be more stable indicators of functional T cell populations in man.

Despite the ambiguities involved in using differential PHA/Con A reactivities as markers for subpopulations of T cells, there are two situations in which preferential mitogen reactivity may be helpful. The first involves human peripheral blood cells reacting to suboptimal concentration of mitogen used (Fig. 2). For both PHA and Con A there is a certain concentration that induces optimal reactivity. Concentrations below (suboptimal) or above (supraoptimal) this elicit substantially less blastogenesis. It can be demonstrated that T cells that bear the Fcγ receptor and thus contain Ts are more responsive to suboptimal PHA than to suboptimal Con A concentrations. At higher mitogen concentrations, Con A is clearly able to activate Ts.

This leads to the second situation in which these T-dependent mitogens have been clinically useful. Net immune reactivity to antigenic stimuli not only requires activation of effector cells, but also depends on the net balance between regulatory influences capable of amplifying or suppressing that reactivity. The chemical structure, dose, and route of administration of the antigen as well as other factors controlled by genes localized to the major histocompatibility locus determine whether Th or Ts will predominate. Advantage has been taken of the fact that mitogens can simulate antigen-induced activation of regulatory T cells. Con A can activate both helper and suppressive T cells, the relative proportion of Th or Ts activated being somewhat dependent on the concentration of Con A utilized. Thus, Con A has been used to activate regulatory T cells occurring among normal peripheral blood mononuclear cells (PBMC) in order to determine afferent and efferent events involved in their biology and to determine the role of regulatory cells

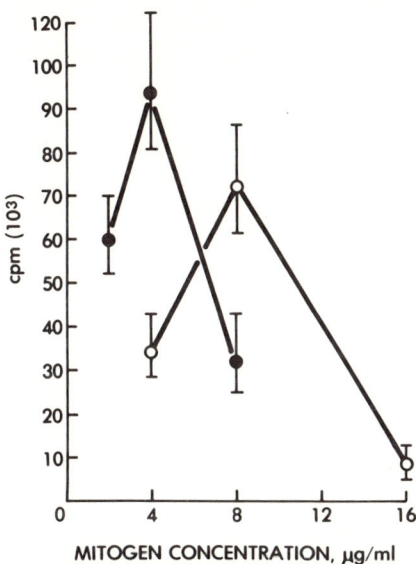

Fig. 2. Dose response curves for phytohemagglutinin (PHA, ●) and concanavalin A (Con A, ○) induced blastogenesis. The indicated final concentrations of either PHA or Con A were used to activate the PBMC from 20 different normals. Reactivity was measured by the incorporation of tritiated thymidine and is expressed as geometric mean counts per minute ± the range encountered by one standard error of the mean. Note the relatively narrow range for maximal mitogen reactivity and the wide variation of reactivity among the 20 different PBMCs.

in the immune dysfunction associated with a variety of clinical disorders. Examples of this will be subsequently presented.

As previously indicated, a relatively large proportion of the progeny derived from lymphocytes activated by PWM are immunoglobulin-secreting plasma cells. However, PWM-induced conversion of B cells into plasma cells is regulated by a balance between Th and Ts cells in a manner analogous to that involved in determining the net amount of specific antibody secreted in response to challenge with antigen. Although it has been possible to generate antigen-induced specific antibody production *in vitro* with murine spleen cells, attempts to reproduce this with human PBMC have met with varied success. However, *in vitro* activation of human PBMC does result in polyclonal Ig production. Utilizing this model, it has been possible to explore intrinsic abnormalities among B cells as well as extrinsic imbalances in T-dependent regulatory influences related to aberrancies of immunoglobulin production associated with several clinical disorders.

Blast transformation induced by mitogens represents the culmination of a complex series of metabolic events that are initiated by suitable perception of the activating signal. This is followed by changes in the alignment and fluidity of cell surface receptors, influx of divalent cations, activation of adenyl cyclase, changes in the intracellular levels of cyclic nucleotides, protein synthesis, RNA synthesis, and, finally, synthesis of new DNA. It is necessary to recognize cell interactions and metabolic events involved in lectin-induced blast transformation in order to understand defects related to decreased mitogen responsiveness associated with clinical disorders. For example, in some disorders characterized by the presence of autoantibodies directed against lymphocytes and monocytes, these antibodies can interfere with cell surface binding of the mitogen or with macrophage T interactions required for full blastogenesis. In other disorders, lymphocytes and macrophages liberate agents (i.e., prostaglandins) that cause elevations in intracellular cyclic AMP. This is perceived by lymphocytes as an "off signal" and can result in decreased mitogen-induced blastogenesis. Finally, it is possible to encounter situations in which *in vitro* lectin-induced blast transformation is markedly deficient, but *in vivo* immune function is remarkably intact. This reflects the fact that many of the immune capabilities of lymphocytes simply require protein synthesis and liberation of lymphokines, but not new DNA synthesis. The regulatory function of Th and the activity of effector T cells participating in reactions of delayed hypersensitivity are good examples of this. Neither of these reactivities requires synthesis of new DNA.

III. Procedure for Determining *in Vitro* Lectin-Induced Activation of Lymphocytes

Assays to measure *in vitro* lectin-induced activation of lymphocytes requires a preparation of lymphocytes and macrophages that is relatively free of contaminating red blood cells, platelets, and granulocytes. These latter cell types do not survive well in culture, and in process of dying they release soluble materials that affect the viability of reactive mononuclear cells. Although several human lymphoid organs (thymus, tonsil, spleen) have been used as a source of lymphocytes, peripheral blood is the most common and accessible. Populations enriched in reactive mononuclear cells are obtained by sedimenting the buffy coat from heparinized (preservative free) peripheral blood over a dense medium of Ficoll–Hypaque. Mononuclear cells (70% T cells, 6% B cells, 20% monocytes–macrophages, <3% granulocytes) remain at the top of the Ficoll–Hypaque while red blood cells, platelets, and granulocytes sediment to the bottom. Usually, approximately 1×10^6 mononuclear cells are obtained for each milliliter of blood drawn.

The actual assay for activation is performed in wells of a microtiter plate. The degree of activation is dependent on the following four variables.

1. The type of serum used in the culture medium. Most laboratories utilize either fetal calf serum (FCS) or pooled AB serum (the serum is heated at 56°C for 0.5 hour to inactivate complement and is diluted to a final concentration of 5–15% in culture medium). Different lots of fetal calf serum vary with regard to their ability to support mitogencsis. In general, lymphocytes cultured in pooled AB serum tend to respond better than do those cultured in FCS. Autologous serum can also be used. However, this introduces another problem related to the tremendous variability among individual sera regarding their affects on lymphocyte proliferation.

2. The density of cells cultured. The complex cellular interactions and cell–cell contact involved in lectin-induced blastogenesis can be dramatically altered simply by changing the density of cells cultured. For example, the reactivity of cells cultured in flat-bottom microtiter wells may be less than that noted when the same number of cells are incubated in round or V-bottom microtiter cells (in the flat-bottom wells, the cells are more dispersed, and thus there is less chance for cell–cell contact). For similar reasons, the degree of blastogenesis is not a direct linear function of the density of cells tested. There exists a minimal density (usually 20,000–50,000 cells per round-bottom microtiter well) required for substantial reactivity. At high cell densities (>150,000 cells per well), nutrients in the culture medium may be depleted, resulting in cell death. These considerations of cell density and interactions apply also to situations in which the reactivity of similar numbers of mononuclear cells containing variable frequencies of T cells, B cells, or monocytes are compared. The net reactivity of a population containing half the normal frequency of T cells may not be 50% of normal.

3. The length of time cells are cultured before activation is assayed.

For PHA and Con A, substantial reactivity (as measured by blast transformation) begins after 2 days of *in vitro* stimulation, peaks at about day 4, and then diminishes. In contrast, maximal blastogenesis and Ig synthesis induced by PWM begins at about day 4 and maximal reactivity occurs 6–7 days after culture. A documented extension of these observations is that T cell reactivity occurs before B cell proliferation. Indeed, the reactivity noted in response to PHA and Con A after day 5 represents that occurring among B cells. In early studies in which PHA or Con A were used to assay reactivity among patients with T cell deficiency, it was noted that the early (day 3–4) response was decreased whereas the late response (day 5–6) was normal. In retrospect, this probably was a reflection of normal or slightly increased frequency of B cells in these patients, rather than an indication of the presence of abnormal, late reacting population of T cells.

4. The concentration of lectin used. The blastogenic response to PHA, Con A, and PWM is dependent on the concentration of mitogen used (while this is in the microgram range, each laboratory has to establish its own dose response curve). Most important, the dose response curve may vary from individual to individual. Thus, if one is comparing maximal mitogen reactivity among different patients and normals, several (usually 3–4) concentrations of mitogens must be used. In many diseases, an apparent decrease in mitogen reactivity simply reflects a shift in the concentration of mitogen required to elicit maximal reactivity.

Determinations used to measure lectin-induced stimulation take advantage of the metabolic changes occurring during activation. Thus, it is possible to measure influx of divalent cations, increases in adenyl cyclase, cyclic AMP, or protein synthesis, as parameters of activation. For clinical studies with Con A and PHA, DNA synthesis or blast transformation are commonly used. For PWM, blast transformation or *in vitro* Ig synthesis are suitable indicators of activation. Blast transformation is assayed either by morphologically counting the frequency of blast cells or by determining the incorporation of a radiolabeled nucleotide (i.e., tritiated thymidine) into newly synthesized DNA. Usually there is a good correlation between these two determinations. However, in some situations in which there is an excess in the frequency of macrophages or a lot of cell death, cold thymidine is released into the culture medium. This competes with the radiolabeled thymidine for incorporation into DNA, thus giving a falsely low indication of blast transformation. Determinations of Ig synthesis utilize either radioimmunoassay or plaque-forming assays capable of measuring the small amounts (nanograms) of total Ig synthesized. As indicated previously, techniques capable of measuring specific antibody formation by PBMC, *in vitro,* have only recently been developed.

There has been much discussion as to how results indicating lectin-induced activation should be presented. One approach is to present data as an index of stimulation (reactivity noted for cells tested in the presence of lectin/baseline or nonstimulated reactivity for cells cultured in the absence of lectin; a small amount of variable "nonstimulated" blastogenesis occurs among the PBMC of all individuals). The problem with this method is that alterations in the stimulation index (SI) could reflect changes in either the numerator or the denominator. For example, an abnormally low SI could reflect either abnormally mitogen-induced reactivity or abnormally high nonstimulated, baseline reactivity.

Another approach has been simply to present either absolute reactivity or absolute minus nonstimulated reactivity (this is usually denoted as change in counts per minute (Δcpm) if reactivity is assayed by the uptake of tritiated thymidine). Antagonists of this approach argue that it does not properly consider relative reactivity.

There is no definitive answer indicating the most correct way to present results of lectin-induced activation. However, one must be wary of data presented only as SI without any discussion or mention of absolute reactivity among stimulated and nonstimulated cultures.

In summary, there are many technical points to be considered when evaluating lectin-induced mitogenesis. Without this consideration, it is difficult to determine whether defects in mitogen reactivity reflect either inherent properties of responsive immunocytes related to *in vivo* immunodeficiency or extrinsic alterations introduced during their *in vitro* culture.

IV. Clinical Usefulness of Lectins

Techniques capable of depicting cell surface markers present on lymphocyte populations in man were not generally available until the early 1970s. Initially, therefore, lectins served as useful probes to assay quantitatively for the frequency of T and B cells. Substantial proliferation in response to PHA or Con A indicated a normal frequency of T cells whereas a brisk proliferative response to PWM reflected an adequate number of B cells. For the most part, PBMC from patients with congenital thymic deficiencies manifested a low response to PHA and to Con A, and those from patients with congenital hypogammaglobulinemia responded poorly to PWM. With the delineation of markers (i.e., sheep red blood cell receptor, surface Ig) useful in quantitating T and B cells, it soon became apparent that defective reactivity to PHA, Con A, or PWM could occur in the presence of a normal frequency of peripheral blood T and B cells. In turn, this suggested that lectin-induced mitogenesis might be subject to regulatory influences similar to those that modulate reactivity to specific antigens. Indeed, lectins are presently utilized not only to explore human immune function *in vitro*, but also to delineate factors capable of modulating immune reactivity.

If lectin-induced blastogenesis is used as an indication of immunological integrity, a crucial question concerns the relevance of *in vitro* blast transformation to *in vivo* immunity. For PWM, this seems clear. Clinically apparent panhypogammaglobulinemia and selective immunoglobulin deficiency correlate with the failure of PWM to induce total or selective Ig synthesis *in vitro*. Moreover, it appears that factors regulating *in vitro* PWM-induced Ig synthesis are similar to those operative in controlling specific antibody production *in vivo*. (It should be emphasized that delineation of these factors, in man, is not complete. It is possible that future work may demonstrate differences between *in vivo* and *in vitro* events.)

The relationship between *in vitro* blastogenesis induced by either PHA or Con A to *in vivo* cell-mediated immunity is less clear. There are clinical situations in which *in vitro* blastogenesis induced by these lectins appears normal in the face of deficient *in vivo* T cell dysfunction, and vice versa. There are several explanations for this. Many T-dependent functions, such as the regulatory function of Th, the cytotoxic ability of killer T cells, and the ability of effector T cells active in delayed hypersensitivity to recruit and activate other mononuclear cells, do not require synthesis on new DNA. Moreover, the polyclonal activation induced by PHA or Con A may actually be a disadvantage for determining subtle immune defects, such as failure to react to a single antigen. In some patients with chronic mucocutaneous candidiasis, for example, there is a deficiency of T cells specifically capable of responding to *Candida albicans*. As this single clone represents only a small portion of the total T cells activated by PHA or Con A, *in vitro* proliferative responses to these mitogens may be only minimally reduced and appear normal. Finally, technical differences among various laboratories in assaying PHA and Con A reactivity have rendered comparisons of responsiveness among a given patient population difficult. In summary, PHA- or Con A-induced blastogenesis is used only as a gross indicator of T cell immunity and should be performed in conjunction with other *in vivo* testing (delayed hypersensitivity skin tests, for example). While a marked deficiency in PHA or Con A reactivity usually is accompanied by some *in vivo* T cell dysfunction, normal or near normal reactivity does not rule out the possibility of a clinically significant abnormality of *in vivo* cell-mediated immunity.

Defects in proliferative reactivity ot PHA, Con A, and PWM have been noted in a variety of disorders ranging from Hodgkin's disease to kwashiorkor. In many instances, abnormal reactivity is accompanied by a diminished frequency of T and B cells. Thus, the defect is related to a quantitative deficiency of potentially responsive cells. However, in many patients, low mitogen reactivity occurs in the presence of normal relative frequencies of responsive mononuclear cells. In these situations there is a qualitative abnormality that prevents substantial blast transformation. Factors related to these qualitative abnormalities are discussed in the following sections (see Table I).

A. Influence of Soluble Serum Factors

The influence of serum factors on immune reactivity is detected by comparing *in vitro* lectin-induced activation among PBMC tested in patients' versus normal serum. Patients' serum can affect reactivity either by lacking as yet undefined soluble materials required to support *in vitro* blast transformation or by containing materials that suppress new DNA synthesis. The latter situation has been more commonly observed, and there are a variety of soluble suppressive materials that may be elevated in many disorders. In some cases, the soluble suppressive materials may actually bind, *in vivo,* to patients' mononuclear cells (α-fetoprotein, antilymphocyte antibodies and immune complexes, for example). In this situation, patients' lymphocytes will exhibit decreased blastogenesis even when cultured in fetal calf or normal serum. These soluble materials can be removed either by incubating the PBMC in FCS or normal serum at 37°C for 2–12 hours prior to testing with lectins (owing to membrane turnover, these materials elute from the cell surface) or by gently treating the cells with proteolytic enzymes capable of cleaving the suppressing material from the cell

TABLE I
EXTRINSIC MECHANISMS RELATED TO DIMINISHED MITOGEN REACTIVITY IN CLINICAL DISORDERS

Mechanism	Disorder
I. Suppressive serum substances[a]: α-fetoprotein, low density lipoprotein, antilymphocyte antibodies, C-reactive protein, etc.	Many, including malignancies, liver and autoimmune diseases, infections
II. Suppressive macrophages	Hodgkin's disease, sarcoidosis, fungal infections
III. Suppressive T cells	Acquired hypogammaglobulinemia, selective IgA deficiency, acquired T cell hypofunction

[a] This includes only a partial list of suppressive materials and associated disorders.

surface. The relevance of many of the suppressive materials to *in vivo* immune dysfunction is conjectural. It should be remembered that many medications can adversely affect *in vitro* blast transformation.

B. Abnormalities at the Level of the Macrophages

Macrophages can secrete a variety of soluble materials capable of modulating T cell blastogenesis. In some patients with Hodgkin's disease, fungal, viral, and mycobacterial infections, sarcoidosis, and collagen vascular disease, decreased T cell blastogenesis is related to some abnormality in adherent (presumably macrophages) cells. Thus, removal of adherent cells from the PBMC paradoxically results in a marked increase in PHA or Con A reactivity. In some cases, it can be demonstrated that these "suppressor macrophages" inhibit reactivity by synthesizing increased amounts of prostaglandins (PGE_2). If PHA or Con A reactivity among patients' PBMC is tested in the presence of indomethacin, an inhibitor of prostaglandin synthesis, normal responses may be noted. The usefulness of indomethacin in reversing *in vivo* T cell dysfunction remains to be determined. In some patients with multiple myeloma, decreased production of normal immunoglobulins appears to be associated with the presence of macrophages capable of inhibiting synthesis of normal Ig but not synthesis of the myeloma immunoglobulin.

Defective T cell blastogenesis may also represent the failure of macrophages to secrete soluble materials required to amplify PHA and Con A reactivity (seen in sarcoidosis, collagen vascular disease). This can be corrected by the addition of a "mitogenic protein" (approximately 15,000 MW) obtained from normal macrophages. Defects represented by the failure of macrophages to appropriately process or present mitogens to T or B cell surfaces have not been described in man.

C. Imbalances in Regulatory T Cells

Defective mitogen reactivity associated with imbalances between Th and Ts have best been studied in patients with hypogammaglobulinemia. While the majority of patients with congenital hypogammaglobulinemia lack substantial numbers of B cells, the frequency of B cells is usually normal in patients with the acquired form of hypogammaglobulinemia. Nonetheless, PBMC from most of these patients fail to synthesize Ig in response to stimulation with PWM. In some patients, this clearly represents an intrinsic abnormality in the B cells. However, in others, the defective conversion of Ig-bearing B cells into Ig-secreting plasma cells reflects an absence of Th or a preponderance of Ts. This can be demonstrated by coculture experiments in which PWM-induced synthesis of Ig is measured among mixtures of either patients' T cells and normal PBMC (Table II). T-dependent suppressive influences specifically capable of inhibiting PWM-induced Ig synthesis may be distinct from those that inhibit PHA or Con A reactivity. Thus, in patients with hypogammaglobulinemia and a predominance of Ts, PHA, and Con A, reactivity may be normal. Several investigators have also demonstrated that some cases of selective IgA deficiency may reflect an imbalance of regulatory T cells that control only the production of IgA.

If defective Ig production and hypogammaglobulinemia can reflect imbalances in regulatory influences, then one might assume that autoantibody production and hypergammaglobulinemia could similarly represent imbalances among Th or Ts. There has been much specu-

TABLE II
COCULTURE EXPERIMENTS INDICATING REGULATORY DEFECTS AMONG T CELLS FROM PATIENTS WITH ACQUIRED HYPOGAMMAGLOBULINEMIA[a]

Source of added regulatory T cells	Source of responder cells	Ig synthesized/10^6 responder cells (ng)
None	Patient No. 1 PBMC	<200
None	Patient No. 2 PBMC	<200
None	Normal PBMC	6552
Patient No. 1	Normal PBMC	<200
Patient No. 2	Normal PBMC	5832
Normal	Patient No. 1	<200
Normal	Patient No. 2	4763

[a] The table represents a series of experiments designed to delineate regulatory abnormalities related to defective immunoglobulin (Ig) production in patients with acquired hypogammaglobulinemia. T cells from the indicated sources were mixed with patient's or normal peripheral blood mononuclear cells (PBMC), and *in vitro* pokeweed mitogen-induced Ig synthesis was assayed. Both patients synthesized little Ig. The defect in patient No. 1 is associated with a predominance of suppressive T cells, as this patient's T cells inhibit Ig synthesis among normal PBMC. The defect in patient No. 2 is related to a relative absence of helper cells and can be corrected by the addition of normal T.

lation, for example, that autoantibody production associated with SLE could occur secondary to a relative deficiency of Ts that normally serve to inhibit Ig synthesis by autoreactive clones of B cells. Although there have been some reports indicating a deficiency of T-dependent influences capable of dampening PWM-induced Ig synthesis in SLE, this has not been a consistent finding.

From experiments performed in animal models, it is clear that cell-mediated reactivity is also subject to regulatory T influences. Some studies indicate that cutaneous anergy and defective *in vitro* reactivity to PHA and to Con A in man may be associated with a predominance of suppressive T cells. However, more studies are required to determine the extent to which this *in vitro* suppression is related to the *in vivo* T cell dysfunction.

Mitogens have proved to be useful in demonstrating qualitative and quantitative lymphocyte defects in man, but three points are worth emphasizing. First, even among patients with a given disease, mechanisms related to the accompanying immune dysfunction may be heterogeneous. For example, we have studied 40 patients with various types of fungal infection and associated *in vivo* defects of cell-mediated immunity. In some patients, the defect is clearly related to a quantitative deficiency of T cells. In others, the frequency of T cells is normal. The associated abnormalities delineated in this group include intrinsic hyporesponsiveness among T cells, the presence of suppressive materials in the serum, increased prostaglandin synthesis by macrophages, and a predominance of suppressive T cells. Second, the relationship of defined immune defects to a given disease, i.e., which is horse and which is cart, have not always been well defined. In some patients, defective PHA or Con A reactivity, irrespective of the causative mechanisms, may simply be a reflection of disease activity rather than a specific disease etiology. Finally, the relationship between *in vitro* phenomena and *in vivo* realities is not clear. Whether a demonstrated imbalance of influences modulating *in vitro* mitogen reactivity has therapeutic potential for correcting *in vivo* immune dysfunction awaits further investigation. Nonetheless, mitogens have proved to be useful probes for indicating potential avenues for the rational manipulation of immune dysfunction associated with many clinical disorders.

The delineation of immunoregulatory abnormalities that affect mitogenesis in disease states has led to an investigation of forces that modulate mitogen reactivity among normals. Recently, it has been possible to demonstrate that normal macrophages can synthesize immunosuppressive prostaglandins. Net synthesis of Ig induced by PWM is regulated by distinct populations of normally occurring Th and Ts. Utilizing Con A, it has been possible preferentially to activate normal Ts capable of inhibiting Ig synthesis and *in vitro* T cell reactivity (Con A-induced Ts that inhibit Ig synthesis appear to be distinct from those capable of suppressing T cell proliferation). These findings support the concept that factors related to defective *in vitro* mitogen reactivity noted in clinical disorders may not simply represent *in vitro* artifacts.

In this chapter the usefulness of only three mitogens in exploring human lymphocyte biology has been discussed. Many other materials exist that are capable of interacting with and activating lymphocytes. The specificity of these for given lymphocyte populations has not been as completely defined, but some—immune complexes, for example—may prove to be more important modulators of lymphocyte activation *in vivo*. Although PHA, Con A, and PWM were not developed to serve as immunological probes, their ability to mimic immune activation has been invaluable in delineating cellular interactions required for immune function in man.

General Reading References

Marx, J. (1977). Looking at lectins: Do they function in recognition processes? *Science* **196**, 1429.
Pelvs, L., and Strausser, H. (1977). Prostaglandins and the immune response. *Life Sci.* **20**, 903.
Rosenstreich, D., and Mized, S. B. (1978). The participation of macrophages and macrophage cell lines in the activation of T lymphocytes by mitogens. *Immunol. Rev.* **40**, 102.
Tomasi, T. B. (1977). Serum factors which suppress the immune response. In "Regulatory Mechanisms in Lymphocyte Recognition" (D. O. Lucas, ed.), p. 219. Academic Press, New York.
Tomasi, T. B. (1977). T and B cells in clinical disorders. *Disease-A-Month* **23**, 2.
Sharon, N. (1977). Lectins. *Sci. Am.* **236**, 108.
Stobo, J. D. (1972). Phytohemagglutinin and concanavalin A: Probes for murine T cell activation and differentation. *Transplant. Rev.* **11**, 60.
Waldman, T., Broder, S., Blaese, R., Durm, M., Blackman, M., and Strober, W. (1974). Role of suppressor T cells in the pathogenesis of common variable hypogammaglobulinemia. *Lancet* **2**, 609.
Waxdal, M. J. (1975). Differential stimulation of murine T and B cell populations by purified mitogens from pokeweed. In "Immune Recognition" (A. S. Rosenthal, ed.), p. 85. Academic Press, New York.
Weksler, M., and Kuntz, M. (1936). Use of mitogens in the evaluation of T-lymphocyte function. In "Clinical Evaluation of Immune Function in Man" (S. Litwin, C. Christian, and G. Siskind, eds.), p. 151. Grune & Stratton, New York.

Natural Killer Cells and Cells Mediating Antibody-Dependent Cytotoxicity against Tumors

RONALD B. HERBERMAN

Laboratory of Immunodiagnosis, National Cancer Institute, Bethesda, Maryland

I. Introduction 73
II. Methods 74
III. Characteristics of NK Cells and Their Relationship to K Cells 77
IV. Specificity of Natural Cytotoxicity 79
V. Factors Affecting Levels of NK and K Cell Activities 82
VI. Possible Clinical Significance of These Effector Cells 84
References 86

I. Introduction

Natural killer (NK) cells represent a recently described member of the armamentarium of cytotoxic effector cells that, in addition to immune cytotoxic T cells, macrophages, and K cells mediating antibody-dependent cell-mediated cytotoxicity (ADCC), can react against tumor cells and some other types of target cells. In contrast to the cells described in other chapters in this volume, NK cells are defined at this time entirely by their functional characteristics, not by any unique cell surface markers. They may just be a subset of a subpopulation of lymphocytes with a particular set of cell surface markers and morphological characteristics and probably represent only a small percentage of the lymphocytes in human peripheral blood. It seems likely, as will be discussed below in detail, that cells with this type of cytotoxic activity are at a particular, early stage of maturation or development, probably within the T cell lineage.

The phenomenon of cytotoxicity of tumor cells and of cultured cell lines derived from tumors by lymphocytes of many normal individuals first became recognized during the course of studies attempting to examine specific cytotoxic activity of lymphocytes of tumor-bearing individuals against their own tumors or against tumors of the same histological or etiological type. It was initially assumed in those studies that lymphoid cells from normal individuals would be unreactive and thus would serve as good baseline controls for comparison. However, it gradually became apparent that lymphocytes of some normal controls were actually more cytotoxic against some target cells than were the tumor-bearing individuals under study. Many investigators first attributed this anomalous control reactivity to a variety of *in vitro* artifacts (see discussion in Herberman and Gaylord, 1973), but it has subsequently been reasonably well established that much or all of this was due to NK cells. These findings have necessitated a reevaluation of supposed disease-related cytotoxic reactivity of cancer patients, with a need to discriminate clearly between the activity of NK cells and of more specific immune effector cells (Herberman and Oldham, 1975).

In the last few years, a number of laboratories have performed extensive studies on NK cells in man and in rodents, and some of these results will be summarized herein. For more details on natural cell-mediated cytotoxicity and on NK cells, the reader might consult a recent, extensive review on this subject (Herberman and Holden, 1978).

II. Methods

Some of the initial observations on NK cell activity, particularly in man, were made in long-term assays of cytotoxicity, either [^{125}I]iododeoxyuridine release assays (Oldham *et al.*, 1973) or visual microcytotoxicity assays (Takasugi *et al.*, 1973). The [^{125}I]iododeoxyuridine release assay is usually performed for 24–48 hours and involves the measurement of lysis of target cells by the percentage of release of isotope that had been incorporated into the DNA of the nuclei. Killing by some normal donors was detected by testing several individuals in each experiment and determining whether the percentage of release of isotope in cultures of target cells with lymphocytes of some donors was significantly higher than that seen with the least reactive donor. The visual microcytotoxicity assays are considerably more complex, involving visual counting of adherent target cells remaining in each microwell at the end of the test. Decreases in cell numbers could be due to cytolysis, inhibition of proliferation of the target cells during the assay, and/or simple loss of adherence of the target cells from the bottom of the well. Most investigators have dealt with the visual microcytotoxicity assays in a qualitative fashion, performing their tests with only one or two effector cell: target cell ratios and scoring their results as positive or negative, depending on whether the number of cells in an experimental group was significantly different ($p < 0.05$) from the control.

In order to characterize the NK cells in detail and to obtain quantitative data rapidly, most investigators have shifted to the use of a short-term, usually 4-hour, chromium-51 release assay. This assay involves the labeling of a suspension of the target cells with sodium [^{51}Cr]chromate. The ^{51}Cr easily enters most cells and binds covalently to intracellular proteins. During the course of a 4-hour assay at 37°C, most or all of the label remains inside a viable, undamaged cell and is released into the medium only upon cell lysis or at least major damage to the cell surface membrane. Therefore the amount of ^{51}Cr in the medium provides a quantitative indication of the number of cells lysed. The main requirement for this short-term assay is the continued availability of a target cell that is quite sensitive to rapid lysis. For clinical studies, many investigators have begun to use the K-562 tissue culture line, derived from the pleural effusion of a patient with chronic myelogenous leukemia in blast crisis. Most normal donors produce a high percentage of ^{51}Cr release at effector:target cell ratios of 50:1 or higher. For studies of NK activity in mice, most investigators now use YAC-1, RL♂1, or RBL-5, which are all tissue culture cell lines of transplantable lymphomas and are quite susceptible to rapid lysis by lymphocytes of normal donors. In general, tissue culture cell lines are more susceptible to NK activity than are *in vivo* passaged tumors, but some mouse and rat ascitic lymphomas have made good target cells.

As will be discussed in detail in Section III, NK cells are in the same lymphocyte subpopulation as K cells mediating antibody-dependent cell-mediated cytotoxicity (ADCC) against tumor cells, and these cells may in fact be the same. Therefore it has become important to also perform assays of ADCC to determine the precise relationship between these two cytotoxic activities. ADCC assays are usually performed with ^{51}Cr-labeled target cells that have been sensitized with IgG antibodies directed against these cells. Lymphoid cells with receptors for a portion of the IgG molecule, designated the Fc portion, can bind to the antibody-coated target cells. With the right combination of Fc receptor-bearing (FcR+) cells and target cells, rapid lysis at 37°C can then result. Several types of cells bear FcR, including a subpopulation of T cells, B cells, and monocytes or macrophages. The type of FcR+ cell capable of lysing antibody-coated target cells is dependent on the type of target cells. Various types of FcR+ cells can lyse certain erythrocyte targets, but only the K cells, in a lymphocyte subpopulation, are able to rapidly lyse mammalian nucleated target cells, usually tumor cells. Therefore most laboratories performing ADCC assays to measure K cell activity use tumor cell lines. For clinical studies, the most commonly used target cells are either the human Chang liver cell line or the mouse P815 mastocytoma, coated with heterologous, usually rabbit, antibodies.

Most assays for human NK and K cell activities are performed with peripheral blood mononuclear cells, usually separated from heparinized whole blood by centrifugation on Ficoll–Hypaque gradients. Human spleen cells have comparable activity, but lymph node, tonsil, or thymus cells have little or no detectable activity against the usual target cells (West *et al.*, 1978). For studies in mice and rats, spleen cells are most frequently used, but, as in the human, peripheral blood lymphocytes also have good activity. Lymph node cells have had variable degrees of reactivity, and thymus cells are usually inactive.

For more extensive characterization of the NK and K cells, it has been necessary to perform a variety of cell separation procedures based on the presence or the absence of certain cell surface markers. Because of the FcR on these cells, it has been possible to enrich or deplete by interaction with IgG antibody–antigen complexes, usually complexes of erythrocytes (E) and rabbit antibodies (A) to the erythrocytes. When such interaction is performed with EA complexes in suspension, rosettes are formed with the FcR+, which then can be selectively pelleted by centrifugation on a Ficoll–Hypaque gradient. Alternatively, the EA or other immune complexes can be attached to plastic dishes and FcR+ cells selectively become attached to the monolayers. The other major type of fractionation performed in studies of NK and K cells is some procedure for separation or depletion of T cells. For human lymphocytes, this is usually done by rosette formation with sheep erythrocytes, since human T cells appear to be the only cell type with receptors for sheep E. For mouse lymphocytes, the main marker for T cells is the theta (θ) or Thy 1 antigen, and mouse T cells can be selectively lysed by treatment with anti-θ plus complement. For all these separation procedures it has been essential to use optimal conditions, since NK and K cells have frequently been found to have receptors with weak binding properties (termed low affinity receptors) or low densities of θ antigen (West *et al.*, 1977, 1978; Kay *et al.*, 1977; Herberman *et al.*, 1978c).

For quantitative determination of the distribution of cytotoxic activity upon cell separation or other treatments, it has generally not been sufficient to compare the percentage of cytotoxicities at a given effector:target cell ratio. This is because of the usual shape of the cytotoxicity dose response curve, with a plateau at high ratios and a rather steep slope at lower ratios. To compare different cell preparations with similar cytotoxicity slopes accurately, it has been quite helpful to calculate lytic units (Cerottini and Brunner, 1971). A lytic unit is defined as the number of cells needed to give a certain percentage of lysis in the linear part of the dose response curve (usually 20–30%). The calculation of lytic units/10^7 cells provides a quantitative relative comparison of the specific activity among various lymphocyte preparations in a test and total lytic units (lytic units/10^7 cells times number of cells in a given fraction) can indicate how the activity in the unseparated cells is distributed among various subpopulations.

III. Characteristics of NK Cells and Their Relationship to K Cells

On the basis of initial cell separation studies, NK cells appeared to be null cells, i.e., lacking characteristic markers of either T cells or B cells. However, by use of optimal conditions for formation of E rosettes with T lymphocytes, most human NK cells were found to have low affinity receptors for E (West *et al.*, 1977). As a recent further confirmation that human NK cells reside in the T cell lineage, treatment with specific anti-T cell sera plus complement caused virtual elimination of cytotoxic activity (Kaplan and Callewaert, 1978). In mice, high levels of NK activity were found in nude, athymic mice, and this seemed to support the non-T cell nature of NK cells. However, it has been recently shown that treatment with high concentrations of anti-θ serum plus complement, or repeated treatments, eliminated most mouse NK activity (Herberman et al., 1978c). Therefore it now appears that mouse NK cells have a low density of θ antigen. Such low density θ+ cells have been described in nude mice and it seems likely that such cells are pre-T cells. To further support the concept that NK cells may be at an early phase of maturation along the T cell lineage, we have found that incubation for 2 hours with some thymic hormone preparations, which are known to cause further differentiation and increased T cell antigen expression, leads to decreased NK activity.

There are as yet no cell surface antigens on NK cells that are unique or particularly characteristic of all cells with this functional activity. Glimcher et al. (1977) found that a mouse anti-thymocyte alloantiserum reacted specifically with NK cells but not with other lymphocytes. However, this reactivity has been weak and in the presence of complement could cause only a partial decrease in NK activity.

Another cell surface marker on NK cells is the FcR. FcR are readily detected on human NK cells, and methods that deplete FcR+ cells result in virtual elimination of NK activity. In mice and rats, NK cells initially appeared to lack FcR. However, when more sensitive depletion procedures were used, more than half of the NK lytic units were removed (Herberman et al., 1977a; Oehler et al., 1978a). The finding of FcR on NK cells of each of the species studied raised questions about the relationship between NK cells and K cells mediating ADCC. One possible explanation for NK activity is that it is produced by K cells which are "armed" with in vivo bound natural antibodies (Koide and Takasugi, 1977) or react against target cells that become coated with antibodies secreted during the in vitro assay (Troye et al., 1977). However, as summarized in Table I and II, extensive studies in my laboratory and in some others have failed to confirm that IgG is involved in natural cell-mediated cytotoxicity. Despite this, the NK and K cells appear to be in the same subpopulation of lymphocytes and share many characteristics (Herberman et al., 1978b), as summarized in Table III. On the basis of experiments in which some target cells sensitive to NK activity were able to inhibit ADCC, it appears that NK and ADCC activities may be mediated by the same cells (Ojo and Wigzell, 1978; Bonnard et al., 1978). It may be that the same cell can produce cytotoxic effects either by interaction with antibody-coated

TABLE I
EVIDENCE AGAINST MEDIATION OF HUMAN NATURAL KILLER (NK) ACTIVITY
AGAINST K-562 BY IgG ANTIBODIES PRODUCED DURING *in Vitro* CULTURE

1. No effect of addition to assay of Fab or F(ab')$_2$ fragments of antihuman IgG reagents
2. No effect of addition to assay of protein A
3. No spontaneous regeneration of NK activity at 37°C within 48 hours after trypsinization
4. No detectable requirement for B cells for generation of NK cells during culture for 6 days

---

target cells via its FcR or with some target cells via separate "NK receptors."

IV. Specificity of Natural Cytotoxicity

An important issue to be considered is the specificity of natural cytotoxicity. Most of the early studies of rodent NK cells utilized leukemia or lymphoma target cells, and it was initially thought that only those cells were sensitive to NK activity. However, as discussed above, many of the initial observations on human NK were made with monolayer cell lines derived from carcinomas. Such data would suggest that NK cells might actually have a wide range of reactivity. This has been confirmed by extensive studies of the susceptibility of a wide variety of cells to NK activity, and the available information is summarized in Table IV. *In vitro* cell lines of tumors have usually been more susceptible to lysis by NK cells, but some *in vivo* tumor cells have also been susceptible. Although it initially appeared that NK reac-

TABLE II
EVIDENCE AGAINST MEDIATION OF HUMAN NATURAL KILLER (NK) ACTIVITY
AGAINST K-562 BY ARMED K CELLS

1. Elution of cytophilic IgG had no effect on NK activity
2. Inability to consistently rearm trypsinized lymphocytes
3. No evidence for natural antibodies in human sera capable of sensitizing K-562 cells for antibody-dependent cell-mediated cytotoxicity
4. No effect of pretreatment of lymphocytes with Fab or F(ab')$_2$ fragments of antihuman IgG reagents

TABLE III
SUMMARY OF SIMILARITIES BETWEEN NATURAL KILLER (NK) AND K CELLS[a]

	Mouse	Human
Effect of age	Absent at birth; peak at 5–9 weeks; then low	Relatively stable
Strain distribution	CBA and nudes high; SJL low	Some donors high, others low
Organ distribution	Activity in blood, spleen, peritoneal cavity, bone marrow; absent in thymus	Activity high in blood and spleen; low in tonsil and lymph node; absent in thymus
Boosting	Rapid increase after LCMV, poly(I:C), interferon	Increase after *in vivo* swine influenza vaccine or poly(I:C) and after interferon *in vitro*
Tumor-bearing	Low activity	Lower activity
T cell markers	Low-density Thy 1 on NK cells; ? also on K cells	Low affinity E-RFC
Fc receptors (FcR)	Detectable with difficulty	Easily detectable
Cell size	Small lymphocyte	Small lymphocyte
Effect of X-ray	Moderately resistant	Marked decrease within 18 hours after 1000 R *in vitro*
In vitro culture	Parallel lability under usual culture conditions and retention of activity under certain conditions	Generation from FcR cells after culture *in vitro* for 4–6 days in medium containing FBS
Cross-inhibition and/or adsorption	Unlabeled NK target cells inhibit ADCC and antibody-sensitized tumor cells inhibit NK activity	K cells adsorbed on cell monolayers removing NK cells, and unlabeled K-562 cells inhibit ADCC

[a] ADCC, antibody-dependent cell-mediated cytotoxicity; E-RFC, cells forming rosettes with sheep erythrocytes; FBS, fetal bovine serum; LCMV, lymphocytic choriomeningitis virus.

tivity was restricted to target cells of the same species, mouse and rat NK cells have been found to have activity against human cell lines (Haller *et al.*, 1977). Reactivity of human NK cells against some rodent target cells appears to occur less frequently. NK activity has also been shown not to be restricted to tumor cells, some types of normal cells having some sensitivity to lysis (Nunn *et al.*, 1977).

Given this rather wide spectrum of reactivity for NK cells, the question then arises whether a single NK receptor reacts rather indiscriminately against all the susceptible target cells or whether there are a variety of NK receptors with specificity for an array of possible an-

TABLE IV
RANGE OF TARGET CELLS SUSCEPTIBLE TO NATURAL KILLER ACTIVITY

1. Leukemias and lymphomas
2. Some sarcomas and carcinomas
    a. Mouse *in vivo* and *in vitro* lines
    b. Human primary tumors and cell lines
3. Some heterologous tumor cells as well as those of same species
4. Some normal cells
    a. Mouse macrophages after adherence for 18 hours
    b. Mouse and human bone marrow cells
    c. Mouse thymus cells
    d. Human thymus cells stimulated with phytohemagglutinin

tigens on target cells. As summarized in Table V, there are several lines of evidence to support the latter possibility, of recognition by NK cells of at least several broad antigenic specificities. Many of the data in this regard were obtained by the cold target inhibition assay. This assay consists of addition of various unlabeled target cells to the mixture of effector cells and ^{51}Cr-labeled target cells. Cells that can interact with the same NK cells mediating lysis of the labeled target cells will

TABLE V
EVIDENCE THAT NATURAL KILLER (NK) CELLS RECOGNIZE AT LEAST SEVERAL BROAD ANTIGENIC SPECIFICITIES

1. In cold target inhibition studies with mouse and human NK cells, patterns of inhibition by various cells vary with labeled target cells
    a. Greatest inhibition usually by same cells used as target
    b. Some targets susceptible to NK are unable to inhibit lysis of other targets
    c. Human acute leukemia cells susceptible to NK but unable to inhibit lysis of K-562
2. Cytotoxicity against heterologous target cells
    a. Susceptibility to lysis by heterologous NK cells varies independently from susceptibility to lysis by NK cells of same species
    b. Human NK cells unreactive against, and not inhibited by, most mouse and rat lines
3. Variation among mouse strains in NK activity against some targets
    a. A/J mice have low activity against most targets, but higher activity against cultured RL♂1 cells
    b. Some strains, but not BALB/c, reactive against RL♂1 ascites cells
4. Leukemia virus gp69/71 inhibits NK of one mouse strain–target cell combination but not others
5. Probable mediation of Hh bone marrow resistance by mouse NK cells

competitively inhibit ^{51}Cr release. When different labeled target cells are used in such studies, varying patterns of inhibition are seen. Some cells that can strongly inhibit lysis of one target have little or no inhibitory activity for other target cells. In addition, there are major differences in the reactivity of NK cells from different mouse strains against some target cells but not against others. Also, in view of the strong parallels between mouse NK cells and the cell mediating *in vivo* bone marrow resistance, it seems likely that NK cells can specifically recognize the genetically determined Hh histocompatibility antigens.

V. Factors Affecting Levels of NK and K Cell Activities

In mice and rats, the levels of NK and K cell activities follow a characteristic age-related pattern. Reactivity first appears at 3–4 weeks of age, reaches peak levels between 5 and 10 weeks of age, and declines to low levels thereafter. There are also considerable differences in levels of activity among various strains (Herberman and Holden, 1978). In man, NK activity is not so clearly age-related, activity being found even in some cord blood samples. However, normal human donors do vary considerably in their levels of reactivity, and some of this has been shown to be genetically linked (Santoli *et al.*, 1976). It has been of considerable interest to determine the mechanisms responsible for the age-related and genetic differences and whether environmental factors may influence these activities. Some clues were initially obtained by observations that inoculation of mice with a variety of viruses, immune adjuvants such as Bacillus Calmette-Guerin or *Corynebacterium parvum*, or tumor cells susceptible to NK activity, could induce a rapid and strong augmentation of reactivity (Herberman *et al.*, 1977b; Wolfe *et al.*, 1976). The finding that rat NK activity could be strongly boosted by poly (I:C) (Oehler *et al.*, 1978b), a potent interferon inducer, raised the possibility that interferon might play a central role in activating NK cells. A variety of interferon inducer have been found to augment NK activity in mice, and inoculation of interferon itself led to boosting of activity within 3 hours (Djeu *et al.*, 1978; Gidlund *et al.*, 1978). Incubation of mouse spleen cells with poly (I:C) or with interferon also has resulted in appreciable increases in NK activity. Similar observations have been made with human NK and K cells (Herberman *et al.*, 1978a,d). Administration of poly (I:C) to some patients resulted in increased levels of cytotoxicity after 2 days. Incubation of human peripheral blood lymphocytes with three different interferon preparations for 1 hour or 18 hours caused increased NK and K cell activities with most donors. The mediation of these effects by interferon has been confirmed in both mouse and human studies by demonstrations that anti-interferon antibodies could eliminate the boosting effect by either the interferon preparations or poly(I:C) (Djeu et al., 1978; Gidlund et al., 1978; Herberman et al., 1987d). In addition, in the human studies the anti-interferon antibodies have caused the levels of NK and ADCC activities to decrease below the spontaneous levels. Such data have suggested that interferon may be important in the spontaneous activation of these effector cells, or at least in the maintenance of their activities.

There has also been considerable interest in conditions or agents that cause decreased NK or K cell activities. In mice and rats, NK cells have been moderately resistant to X-irradiation, but at least in our studies high doses have caused appreciable decreases in activity. Cyclophosphamide and hydrocortisone have been found to have strong inhibitory effects. In contrast to the inhibitory effect on NK cells, boosting of NK by poly(I:C) is unaffected by X-irradiation or by these drugs. It appears that the NK cells differentiate from a more resistant precursor (Oehler and Herberman, 1978). It is of note that macrophage toxic agents, carrageenan and silica, have also decreased NK activity in rodents. This appears to be due to the important role of macrophage in producing interferon and thereby activating NK cells.

In contrast to the inhibitory effects of some immunosuppressive agents, NK activity remains normal or elevated in most immunodeficiency diseases. Athymic nude mice, CBA/N mice with defective B cell responses, and even athymic asplenic mice, with combined T and B cell deficits, have high levels of NK activity. Patients with agammaglobulinemia have also been found usually to have normal levels of NK activity (Koren et al., 1978; Pross et al., 1979). This would appear to be another line of evidence against an important role for IgG in NK activity. Perhaps analogous to nude mice, a patient with thymoma and depressed T cell functions had high NK activity. There is some controversy over the levels of K cell activity in patients with agammaglobulinemia, with one report indicating low or absent levels (Koren et al., 1978) while another found this function to be intact (Pross et al., 1978). The reasons for this major discrepancy are not clear, but they may be related to the different target cells used in each study.

VI. Possible Clinical Significance of These Effector Cells

One of the most important questions to be answered about NK and K cells is what role they play *in vivo*. Of particular concern is whether they represent an important defense mechanism against tumor growth or microbial infections. This is very difficult to determine in man, and we must rely heavily on evidence in animal systems. Such an extrapolation would appear to be justified, since most major characteristics of human, mouse, and rat NK and K cells have been found to be quite comparable. Unfortunately, however, even in syngeneic mouse or rat systems, conclusive evidence is very difficult to obtain. This is largely due to the current inability to selectively deplete only NK and/or K cells or to obtain a pure population of these cells to transfer into recipients with low or absent activity. It has been possible to design experiments in which mature T cells would play little or no role, but it has been more difficult to discriminate between NK cells, K cells, and macrophages.

Most of the currently available evidence for an *in vivo* role of mouse NK cells is based on various types of correlations with *in vitro* observations (Herberman and Holden, 1978) (Table VI). Although none of these observations is sufficiently compelling, taken together they strongly suggest that NK cells can under at least some circumstances play an important role in resistance against tumor growth. The recent findings on the role of interferon in activating NK cells, and the im-

TABLE VI
Evidence for *in Vivo* Role of Natural Killer (NK) Cells

1. Poor growth of some NK-sensitive tumors in nude mice
2. Fewer transplantable tumors induced in mice 5–10 weeks old, at the peak of NK activity, than in older mice
3. Correlation between NK activity and resistance to growth of an NK-sensitive tumor in various strains of mice
4. Close parallels between NK activity and genetically determined (Hh) bone marrow resistance in mice
5. Close parallels between NK activity and radioresistant inhibition of tumor growth in mice
6. High NK activity and increased resistance to tumor growth produced by transfer of bone marrow precursor cells from high NK strains to lethally irradiated low NK strain

portant accessory role that macrophages play in this regard, should help in designing more definitive experiments.

There have been similar problems with establishing the *in vivo* role of K cells and of ADCC. A number of experiments have demonstrated that transfer of serum has a protective effect. However, it is very difficult to distinguish between ADCC and some direct effects of antibodies, especially if those effects might be complement independent.

The original formulations of the theory of immune surveillance focused on the central role of the immune response as a natural defense against neoplasia. Only more recently has the theory been modified to stress the relationship of thymus-dependent immunity to immune surveillance. It is this modification of the theory that has aroused a series of criticisms of the concept of immune surveillance, and even led to a counter theory of immune stimulation. Much attention has been directed toward two apparent contradictions to the theory of immune surveillance—the relatively low incidence of tumors in nude mice and the failure of some tumors to develop in thymectomized mice. Although these data do challenge the modified concept of immune surveillance, in which thymus-dependent immunological reactions are required for effective antitumor resistance, they do not really bear on the basic theory itself. The discovery that nude mice and neonatally thymectomized mice and rats have high levels of NK and ADCC activities, potentially very effective alternative mechanisms for immune surveillance, provides a good explanation for most of the available *in vivo* data.

The available information on the incidence of tumors in immunodeficient or immunosuppressed humans has also engendered controversy regarding the role of immune surveillance. With some forms of depressed immunity, the incidence of some types of tumors, especially those of the reticuloendothelial system, have been clearly increased. However, in other diseases associated with immune depression, e.g., leprosy, an increased incidence of cancer has not been noted. As discussed earlier, this variable association of immune depression with elevated tumor incidence might be related to different effects of disease or immunosuppressive regimen on NK and ADCC activities and other possible defense mechanisms. It will be very important to evaluate carefully the levels of these effector functions in the various conditions and to determine whether any correlate with the incidence of tumors in these patients.

The other principal challenge to the concept of immune surveillance has been that, in contrast to the antigenicity of virus-induced tumors, spontaneous tumors frequently lack detectable antigenicity and therefore might not be susceptible to control by the immune system. Much has been made of the findings that tumors arising *in vitro* are not more antigenic than those arising *in vivo*, where the immune system might have been expected to select for tumors with weak or absent tumor-associated antigens. However, almost all the negative evidence has been obtained by procedures designed to detect transplantation resistance and other immune responses that generally have been associated with immune T cell activity. If, as suggested here, there is a role for NK and K cells in immune surveillance, then the question of antigenicity and resistance to tumor growth needs to be asked by protocols designed to detect this function as well as that of immune T cell-mediate cytotoxicity.

References

Bonnard, G. D., Kay, H. D., Herberman, R. B. , Ortaldo, J. R., Djeu, J., Pfiffner, K. J., and Oehler, J. R. (1978). Models for the mechanism of natural cell-mediated cytotoxicity. I. Relationship to antibody-dependent cell-mediated cytotoxicity. In "Prospective in Immunology" (G. Riethmuller, P. Wernet, and G. Cudkowicz, eds.). Academic Press, New York.
Cerottini, J.-C., and Brunner, K. T. (1971). *In vitro* assay of target cell lysis by sensitized lymphocytes. In "*In Vitro* Methods in Cell-Mediated Immunity" (B. R. Bloom and P. R. Glade, eds.), pp. 369–373. Academic Press, New York.
Djeu, J. Y., Heinbaugh, J. A., Holden, H. T., and Herberman, R. B. (1978). Augmentation of mouse natural killer cell activity by interferon and interferon inducers. *J. Immunol.* **122,** 175–181.
Gidlund, M., Örn, A., Wigzell, H., Senik, A., and Gesser, I. (1978). Enhanced NK cell activity in mice injected with interferon and interferon inducers. *Nature (London)*.
Glimcher, L., Shen, F. W., and Cantor, H. (1977). Identification of a cell-surface antigen selectively expressed on the natural killer cell. *J. Exp. Med.* **145,** 1–9.
Haller, O., Kiessling, R., Örn, A., Kärre, K., Nilsson, K., and Wigzell, H. (1977). Natural cytotoxicity to human leukemia mediated by mouse non-T cells. *Int. J. Cancer* **20,** 93–103.
Herberman, R. B., and Gaylord, C. E., eds. (1973). Conference and workshop on cellular immune reactions to human tumor-associated antigens. *Natl. Cancer Inst. Monogr.* **37,** 1–221.
Herberman, R. B., and Holden, H. T. (1978). Natural cell-mediated immunity. *Adv. Cancer Res.* **27,** 305–377.
Herberman, R. B., and Oldham, R. K. (1975). Problems associated with study of cell-mediated immunity to human tumors by microcytotoxicity assays. *J. Natl. Cancer Inst.* **55,** 749–753.

Herberman, R. B., Bartram, S., Haskill, J. S., Nunn, M. E., Holden, H. T., and West, W. H. (1977a). Fc receptors on mouse effector cells mediating natural cytotoxicity against tumor cells. *J. Immunol.* **119**, 322–326.

Herberman, R. B., Nunn, M. E., Holden, H. T., Staal, S., and Djeu, J. Y. (1977b). Augmentation of natural cytotoxic reactivity of mouse lymphoid cells against syngeneic and allogeneic target cells. *Int. J. Cancer* **19**, 555–564.

Herberman, R. B., Djeu, J. Y., Ortaldo, J. R., Holden, H. T., West, W. H., and Bonnard, G. D. (1978a). Role of interferon in augmentation of natural and antibody-dependent cell-mediated cytotoxicity. *Cancer Treatment Rep.* **62**, 1893–1896.

Herberman, R. B., Holden, H. T., West, W. H., Bonnard, G. D., Santoni, A., Nunn, M. E., Kay, H. D., and Ortaldo, J. R. (1978b). Cytotoxicity against tumors by NK and K cells. *In* "Proceedings of International Symposium on Tumor Associated Antigens and Their Specific Immune Response" (F. Spreafico and R. Arnon, eds.), pp. 129–150. Academic Press, London.

Herberman, R. B., Nunn, M. E., and Holden, H. T. (1978c). Lower density of Thy 1 antigen on mouse effector cells mediating natural cytotoxicity against tumor cells. *J. Immunol.* **121**, 304–309.

Herberman, R. B., Ortaldo, J. R., and Bonnard, G. D. (1978d). Augmentation by interferon of human natural and antibody-dependent cell-mediated cytotoxicity. *Nature* **277**, 221–223.

Kaplan, J., and Callewaert, D. M. (1978). Expression of human T-lymphocyte antigens by natural killer cells. *J. Natl. Cancer Inst.* **60**, 961–964.

Kay, H. D., Bonnard, G. D., West, W. H., and Herberman, R. B. (1977). A functional comparison of human Fc-receptor-bearing lymphocytes active in natural cytotoxicity and antibody-dependent cellular cytotoxicity. *J. Immunol.* **118**, 2058–2066.

Koide, Y., and Takasugi, M. (1977). Determination of specificity in natural cell-mediated cytotoxicity by natural antibodies. *J. Natl. Cancer Inst.* **59**, 1099–1106.

Koren, H. S., Amos, D. B., and Buckley, R. H. (1978). Natural killing in immunodeficient patients. *J. Immunol.* **120**, 796–799.

Nunn, M. E., Herberman, R. B., and Holden, H. T. (1977). Natural cell-mediated cytotoxicity in mice against non-lymphoid tumor cells and some normal cells. *Int. J. Cancer* **20**, 381–387.

Oehler, J. R., and Herberman, R. B. (1978). Natural cell-mediated cytotoxicity in rats. III. Effects of immunopharmacologic treatments on natural reactivity and on reactivity augmented by polyinosinic–polycytidylic acid. *Int. J. Cancer* **21**, 221–229.

Oehler, J. R., Lindsay, L. R., Nunn, M. E., and Herberman, R. B. (1978a). Natural cell-mediated cytotoxicity in rats. I. Tissue and strain distribution, and demonstration of a membrane receptor for the Fc portion of IgG. *Int. J. Cancer* **21**, 204–209.

Oehler, J. R., Lindsay, L. R., Nunn, M. E., Holden, H. T., Herberman, H. T., and Herberman, R. B. (1978b). Natural cell-mediated cytotoxicity in rats. II. *In vivo* augmentation of NK-cell activity. *Int. J. Cancer* **21**, 210–220.

Ojo, E., and Wigzell, H. (1978). Natural killer cells may be the only cells in normal mouse lymphoid populations endowed with cytolytic ability for antibody-coated tumor target cells. *Scand. J. Immunol.* **7**, 297–306.

Oldham, R. K., Siwarski, D., McCoy, J. L., Plata, E. J., and Herberman, R. B. (1973). Evaluation of a cell-mediated cytotoxicity assay utilizing ^{125}iododeoxyuridine-labelled tissue-culture target cells. *Natl. Cancer Inst. Monogr.* **37**, 49–58.

Pross, H. F., Gupta, S., Good, R. A., and Baines, M. G. (1979). Spontaneous human lymphocyte-mediated cytotoxicity against tumor target cells. VII. The effect of immunodeficiency disease. *Cell Immunol.* **43,** 160–167.

Santoli, D., Trinchieri, G., Zmijewski, C. M., and Koprowski, H. (1976). HLA-related control of spontaneous and antibody-dependent cell-mediated cytotoxic activity in humans. *J. Immunol.* **117,** 765–770.

Takasugi, M., Mickey, M. R., and Terasaki, P. I. (1973). Reactivity of normal lymphocytes from normal persons on cultured tumor cells. *Cancer Res.* **33,** 2898–2902.

Troye, M., Perlmann, P., Pape, G. R., Spiegelberg, H. L., Naslund, I., and Gidlof, A. (1977). The use of Fab fragments of anti-human immunoglobulin as analytic tools for establishing the involvement of immunoglobulin in the spontaneous cytotoxicity to cultured tumor cells by lymphocytes from patients with bladder carcinoma and from healthy donors. *J. Immunol.* **119,** 1061–1067.

West, W. H., Cannon, G. B., Kay, H. D., Bonnard, G. D., and Herberman, R. B. (1977). Natural cytotoxic reactivity of human lymphocytes against a myeloid cell line: characterization of effector cells. *J. Immunol.* **118,** 355–361.

West, W. H., Boozer, R. B., and Herberman, R. B. (1978). Low affinity E-rosette formation by the human K cell. *J. Immunol.* **120,** 90–95.

Wolfe, S. A., Tracey, D. E., and Henney, C. S. (1976). Induction of "natural killer" cells by BCG. *Nature (London)* **262,** 584–586.

Regulation of the Immune System by Lymphocyte Sets: Analysis in Animal Models

H. CANTOR

*Harvard Medical School/Farber Cancer Institute,
Harvard University, Boston, Massachusetts*

I. General Considerations	89
II. Analysis in the Mouse	91
III. Conclusions	95
Selected References	97

I. General Considerations

The important cells in the immune system are lymphocytes and macrophages. Macrophages line the tissues of the body, ingest foreign material, and present it to lymphocytes. Lymphocytes circulate freely through the blood and lymphatic vessels of the body and bear clonally distributed receptors for antigen. Lymphocytes are directly responsible for all specific immune responses. They are divisible into two sorts: (*a*) the T lymphocytes (or T cells), so-called because their maturation requires processing in the thymus; and (*b*) the B lymphocytes (or B cells), which, in mammals, probably are generated mainly in bone marrow.

It should be emphasized that although the field of immunology began at the turn of the century, identification of the lymphocyte as the immunological cell was clearly established only 15–20 years ago. This means that cellular immunology is an extraordinarily young discipline, and that a coherent view of the cellular basis of the immune response is only just beginning to emerge. Until recently, immunologists generally held that the immune system was comprised of clones of lymphocytes that, when activated by antigen, would produce antibody or initiate a cell-mediated response (such as an inflammatory response). According to this view, the duration and strength of a response depends only upon the number of lymphocyte clones in the host that carried receptors for a particular antigen; absence of immunity to "self"-antigens reflects deletion at birth of those clones of lymphocytes bearing receptors for self-antigens.

Over the past decade, increasing evidence has accumulated that this view of the immune system is incorrect. A more accurate description of the immune system is (*a*) it is composed of many sets of regulatory lymphocytes that respond mainly to signals generated from within the system itself and that for the most part these interactions inhibit both antibody and cellular immune responses; and (*b*) that these interactions also serve to prevent "B" lymphocytes from producing antibody against host antigens. In other words, the absence of autoimmune reactions may be due in part to continuous and active suppression rather than the absence of self-reactive cells within the system.

One approach that has supported this view of the immune system involves the dissection and definition of sets of T and B lymphocytes and analysis of the various immune functions that they perform. Despite their uniform morphology, T cells are not a homogeneous population; they comprise subclasses or sets of lymphocytes with different and even seemingly opposing functions. Thus one property of T cells, called helper function, is to assist B cells to make antibody. A second function of T cells had been suspected from investigations of immunological tolerance or unresponsiveness. These studies indicated that the adoptive transfer of T lymphocytes from an animal unresponsive to a given antigen to a normal animal could render the recipient specifically unresponsive. This property of T cells has been termed "suppressor" function and has been subsequently observed in a large number of immunological experiments. At some risk of oversimplification, it is likely that suppressor function is a necessary homeostatic control mechanism that keeps the immune system of individuals "in trim" and prevents untoward autoimmune reactions. Another property of T cells is the generation of cells that are capable of damaging or destroying cells recognized as antigenically foreign after, for example, infection by a virus. This is associated with cytotoxic or killer function of T cells. Yet another function of T cells involves the ability of these cells to induce or activate other cells to participate in inflammatory responses.

A crucial point arises: Are all these functions invested in a *single* set of T cells that have differentiated in the thymus, and are these diverse responses governed entirely by extraneous conditions, such as a mode or type of antigen stimulation? Alternatively, are these immunological functions invested in distinct sets of T cells that have been programmed to respond in different ways during their differentiative history?

II. Analysis in the Mouse

In the mouse, this question has resolved itself into the practical problem of finding out whether it is possible to subdivide the T cell population into different sets that, when confronted with antigens, are able to make only one or another of the possible T cell responses. At the present time, the most effective technique for identifying and separating subpopulations of peripheral T cells has come from studies of the cell surface components, which become expressed on cells undergoing thymus-dependent differentiation. This classification is based upon the use of alloantisera developed by Boyse and his colleagues that define a pattern of cell surface differentiation components expressed on T cells. Since these components have not been detected on cells of other tissues, such as brain, kidney, liver, or epidermal cells, they are evidently specified by genes expressed *exclusively* during T cell differentiation. These have been called the Lyt systems. The Lyt1 component is coded for by a gene on chromosome 19, and the Lyt2, 3 components are both coded for by genes on chromosome 6. These last two are treated together tentatively because the two genes are tightly linked and these two systems have not so far exhibited any differences other than the fact that genetically they are coded for by distinguishable loci.

In general, the approach involves a cytotoxicity assay similar to the complement-dependent hemolytic test used to identify markers on red cells. As with hemolysis by anti-erythrocyte antibody and complement, lymphocytes exposed to, say, anti-Ly1 sera in the presence of complement are lysed. This lysis can be monitored by the use of trypan blue, which stains lysed but not living, cells or by the release of a radioactive label from the lysed cells. The specificity of this reaction is confirmed by the absence of lysis of cells from "genetically identical" mice that differ only at the relevant *Ly* allele. More recently, these antisera to Lyt1 or Lyt2 components have been used to select "positively" cells bearing these components: columns containing beads that have been coated with anti-Ly1 or anti-Ly2 selectively retain lymphocytes expressing the relevant Ly surface component.

Analysis of this sort has revealed that the peripheral T cell pool contains *at least* three separate T cell sets. We refer to them in shorthand as the Ly123 set, the Ly1 set, and the Ly23 set. They compose, respectively, 50%, 30%, and approximately 10% of the peripheral T cell pool. These findings indicate that, according to the criterion of selective expression of gene products on the cell surface, the T cell pool is divisible into three groups of cells, each following a different set of genetic instructions. The question then becomes whether these individual differentiative programs include information that decides what the function of each T cell set should be. Evidence to date indicates that cells of the Ly1 set are genetically programmed to help or amplify activity of other cells after stimulation by antigen. Ly1 cells are most aptly called *"inducer"* cells, since they will induce or activate other cell sets to fulfill their respective genetic programs: Ly1 cells induce B cells to secrete antibody; they induce macrophages and monocytes to participate in delayed-type hypersensitivity responses: they can, under appropriate circumstances, induce precursors of killer cells to differentiate to killer-effector cells; most recently, and perhaps of most importance, it has been found that Ly1 cells also induce a set of resting, nonimmune T cells to generate potent "feedback" suppressive activity. Analysis of isolated Ly1 inducer cells from nonimmune donors indicates that these cells are already programmed for helper/inducer function *before* overt immunization with antigen; this function is independent of the ability of Ly1 inducer cells to interact with antigen.

By contrast, cells of the Ly23 set are specially equipped to develop both alloreactive cytotoxic activity as well as to suppress both humoral and cell-mediated immune responses. Whether cytotoxicity and suppression are two manifestations of one genetic program or whether they represent the phenotype of two separate genetic programs is not yet established.

It is of particular interest that both sets of T cells see "antigen" in association with the host's own major histocompatibility complex (MHC) gene products: it is likely that these cells are most efficiently activated by antigen (such as a virus) that is associated with MHC products on the surface of living cells. Ly1 cells selectively bind to and are activated by the so-called *I*-region products products of the MHC complex, which corresponds to the HLA-D region products in man. *I*-region products may be recognized as "foreign" either owing to polymorphic variation (alloantigens) or after modification by foreign antigens such as a virus. By contrast, Ly23 cells bind to and react against *H2-KD* gene products of the MHC complex, which roughly correspond to HLA-A and B antigens in man. Thus, the genetic program of these two cell sets appear to include differential reactivity to modified MHC products.

Proof that these two cell sets, which are marked by different surface Ly phenotypes and different functional potentials, in fact represent two branches of thymus-directed differentiation comes from experiments in which isolated Ly1 cells and Ly23 cells are used to repopulate the lymphoid tissues of mice that have been depleted of their T cell system. These recipients lack detectable numbers of T cells and are called B mice. Recipients of Ly1 cells have been called B-Ly1 mice, and recipients of Ly23 cells have been called B-Ly23 mice. For as long as we have observed them, B-Ly1 mice are equipped for helper function but not killer function; B-Ly23 mice express killer but not helper function. These findings show that Ly1 and Ly23 cells have already exercised differentiative options that prevent them from giving rise to one another. In other words, these two T cell sets belong to different lines of differentiation and are not sequential stages of a single progression.

Until recently, cells of the Ly123 set have been the least well defined of the various T cell sets. The most likely possibility is that at least some Ly123 cells represent a store of receptor-positive intermediary cells that regulate the supply and function of more mature Ly1 and Ly23 cells. This is based in part on (*a*) experiments showing that after stimulation with virus-infected syngeneic cells, some Ly123 cells give rise to Ly23 progeny; and (*b*) experiments indicating that purified populations of Ly123 cells can give rise to Ly1 cells after polyclonal activation by concanavalin A. That at least a portion of Ly123 cells represent a precursor pool is also consistent with earlier observations that cells of the Ly123 subclass are detectable in the spleens of mice within the first week of life, whereas both Ly1 and Ly23 cells do not reach maximal numbers until adult life (8–12 weeks of age).

More recently, it has been demonstrated that antigen-stimulated Ly1 cells, or supernatants of activated Ly1 cells, in addition to inducing B cells to secrete antibody, can induce or activate resting Ly123 T cells to develop profound "feedback" suppressive activity. Feedback suppression is appropriate here since the degree of suppressive activity exerted by a fixed number of nonimmune Ly123 cells increases in direct proportion to the numbers of antigen-activated Ly1 cells in the system. This Ly1–Ly123 interaction has also been shown to influence the immune response *in vivo* in mice and may well represent cell interaction that governs the duration and intensity of immune reactions: after stimulation of the immune system by foreign materials, activated antigen-specific Ly1 cells induce B cells to form antibody and also induce resting Ly123 cells to inhibit T helper cell activity. Reduction in T helper activity is accompanied by decreased induction of B cells as well as progressively decreasing induction of resting Ly123 cells; the net result is progressive decrease in both antibody formation and suppressor cell induction. These findings also indicate that, like the formation of antibody, the generation of immunological suppression after stimulation by antigen is not an autonomous function; both require induction by Ly1 cells.

These negative feedback circuits suggest also that the response to any given antigen may reflect in part the amount of feedback inhibition generated after exposure to that antigen. The response to many antigens is regulated by MHC-linked genes. Each inbred strain of mouse, for example, will not respond to a certain proscribed list of antigens. In some cases, this lack of response reflects exaggerated induction of feedback inhibitory cells that mask delivery of the T-helper signal to the B cell.

These findings suggest that an essential component that regulates both the intensity and type of the immune response involves the ability of Ly1 inducer cells to activate various effector cell systems, on the one hand, as well as suppressive systems on the other. It therefore has become critically important to know whether cells of the Ly1 set that induce suppressive activity represent a specialized subgroup of Ly1 cells that differ from cells that, for example, induce B cells to produce antibody. A direct approach to this question has come from the finding that a portion of Ly1 cells also express a newly defined antigen called

Qal. This antigen, or antigen system, is coded for by genes that map between *H2-D* and the *TL* locus of the mouse. Studies of Ly1:Qal$^+$ cells have shown that these cells are responsible for induction of feedback inhibition and that Ly1:Qal$^-$ cells are not. In addition, these studies show that signals from both Ly1:Qal$^+$ and Ly1:Qal$^-$ cells are required for optimal formation of antibody by B cells. Thus the ability of antigenic determinants to induce a detectable antibody response may depend largely on the ratio of Ly1:Qal$^+$ and Ly1:Qal$^-$ T cell clones that bear receptors for that antigen. Recent work has also suggested that the ability of Ly1:Qal$^+$ inducer cells to elicit strong suppressive responses is likely to be particularly important in governing the duration and intensity of inflammatory reactions, such as delayed-type hypersensitivity and IgE-mediated hypersensitivity. Thus analysis of the cell-free products of homogeneous populations of Ly1:Qal$^+$ cells is currently of intense interest, since these materials may well prove to be useful in strategies designed to selectively suppress hypersensitivity or antibody responses to defined antigens.

Analysis of the relative contributions of these T cell sets to an immune response supports the following view: the intensity and specificity of the immune response is determined primarily by interactions among these T cell sets. Specifically, that perturbation of the immune system by antigen results in stimulation of two distinct helper or inducer T cell sets; both deliver signals that activate B cells to produce antibody, but only one activates the T-suppressive system, and it is the strength of this latter interaction that ultimately sets the level and the duration of an immune response.

III. Conclusions

In sum, these experiments have established that the genetic program for a single differentiated set of cells, in this case immunological cells, combines information coding for a surface antigenic profile that is associated with particular physiological functions. Second, they have indicated that the majority of T cells are not effector cells poised to respond to foreign antigen, but regulatory cells that respond mainly to signals or messages generated from within the T cell system itself, and that detectable immune responses reflect perturbations of these signals after the Ly1 system is stimulated by "antigen." The net effect of these T–T interactions after perturbation by antigen is to restore the homeostatic balance of the system, usually at a new level reflecting differentiation of antigen-specific T and B cell clones belonging to the sets described above.

We have just begun to delineate the circuits involved in this regulatory system as summarized above. At the risk of oversimplification, the picture that is beginning to emerge is that Ly1 cells act as sentinel cells that screen the surfaces of other cells, particularly macrophages for foreign material, associated with MHC molecules. When activated, these sentinel cells can induce a variety of effector cells (e.g., B cells that make antibody or macrophages and monocytes that participate in inflammatory responses) to make a specific immune response. In addition, they activate a "committee" of resting T cells that are probably relatively immature. (The term committee is used here because it is virtually certain that Ly123 cells are themselves a heterogeneous set, and perhaps not the sole members of this system. Moreover, the response of a committee is generally suppressive.) This committee of cells emits inhibitory signals. The intensity of inhibition depends mainly on the genetic background of the host, the nature of the antigenic stimulus, and the intensity of the inducing signal emitted by the sentinel cells. The observed immune response depends upon the relative potency and timing of feedback suppressive inhibitory signals.

What happens when this system goes wrong? There are, so far, several animal models that manifest disorders of this immunoregulatory circuit; NZB mice spontaneously develop an autoimmune disorder characterized by the production of a variety of autoantibodies and a clinical syndrome resembling human systemic lupus erythematosus. The major T cell deficit of NZB mice is the absence or malfunction of an Ly123 T cell set responsible for feedback inhibition.

A second example comes from experiments in which $Ly2^+$ regulatory cells are deliverately eliminated from the host: mice depleted of all T cells are repopulated with either Ly1 inducer cells or all T cell sets (including $Ly2^+$ regulatory cells). Within the first 2 weeks after repopulation, sera from the former, but not the latter, mice contain autoantibodies against erythrocytes and thymocytes. Thus, elimination of regulatory T cells that participate in feedback inhibition can be directly shown to result in the formation of autoantibodies.

It should be emphasized that a number of critical questions remain to be answered. Are feedback inhibitory interactions among T cell sets responsible, in part, for self-tolerance beginning at birth? What is the molecular basis underpinning communication among these T cell sets? And, finally, how can we use this information to improve our understanding and treatment of autoimmune disorders in man? No one can say with certainty whether these new insights into the working of the immune system will have an important impact upon treatment of autoimmune disorders in man. Dissection of regulatory T cell circuits is currently the subject of intense experimentation and debate. And perhaps this is the most hopeful and encouraging aspect of this new phase of immunobiology.

Selected References

Alter, B. J., and Bach, F. H. (1974). Role of H-2 lymphocyte defined and serologically defined components in the generation of cytotoxic lymphocytes. *J. Exp. Med.* **140,** 1410.

Bach, F. H., Bach, M. L., and Sondel, P. M. (1976). Differential function of major histocompatibility complex antigens and T lymphocyte activation. *Nature (London)* **259,** 273.

Boyse, E. A., and Old, L. J. (1969). Some aspects of normal and abnormal cell surface genetics. *Annu. Rev. Genet.* **3,** 269.

Broder, S., Humphrey, R., Durm, M., Blackman, M., Meade, B., Goldman, C., Strober, W., and Waldmann, T. A. (1975). Impaired synthesis of polyclonal immunoglobulins by circulating lymphocytes from patients with multiple myeloma. *N. Engl. J. Med.* **293,** 887.

Chess, L., and Schlossman, S. F. (1977). *Adv. Immunol.* **25,** 125–213.

Cantor, H. and Boyse, E. A., (1977). Regulation of cellular and humoral immunity by T cell subclasses. *Cold Spring Harbor Symp. Quant. Biol.* **41,** 23.

Cantor, H., and Weissman, I. (1976). Development and function of subpopulations of thymocytes and T cells. *Prog. Allergy* **20,** 1.

Cantor, H., McVay-Boudreau, L., Hugenberger, J., Naidorf, K., Shen, F. W., and Gershon, R. K. (1978). Immunoregulatory circuits among T-cell sets. II. Physiologic role of feedback inhibition in vivo: absence in NZB mice. *J. Exp. Med.* **147,** 1116.

Dickler, H. B., and Kunkel, H. G. (1972). Interaction of aggregated gammaglobulin with B lymphocytes. *J. Exp. Med.* **136,** 191.

Eardley, D. D., Hugenberger, J., McVay-Boudreau, L., Shen, F. W., Gershon, R. K., and Cantor, H. (1978). Immunoregulatory circuits among T cell sets. I. T-helper cells induce other T-cell sets to exert feedback inhibition. *J. Exp. Med.* **147,** 1106.

Engleman, E. G., McMichael, A. J., Batey, M. E., and McDevitt, H. O. (1978). A suppressor T cell of the mixed lymphocyte reaction in man specific for the stimulating alloantigen. *J. Exp. Med.* **147,** 137.

Evans, R. L., Breard, J. M., Lazarus, H., Schlossman, S. F., and Chess, L. (1977). Detection, isolation and functional characterization of two human T cell subclasses bearing unique differentiation antigens. *J. Exp. Med.* **145,** 2221.

Evans, R. L., Lazarus, H., Penta, A. C., and Schlossman, S. F. (1978). Two functionally distinct subpopulations of human T cells that collaborate in the generation of cytotoxic cells responsible for cell-mediated lympholysis. *J. Immunol.* **120,** 1423.

Good, R. A. (1973). Immunodeficiency in developmental perspective. *Harvey Lec.* **67**, 1.
Gershon, R. K. (1974). T cell suppression. *Comtemp. Topics Immunobiol.* **3**, 1.
Möller, G., ed. (1977). "Immunology and Differentiaiton" (*Immunol. Rev.* **33**). Munksgaard, Copenhagen.
Moretta, L., Ferrarini, M., Mingari, M. C., Moretta, A., and Webb, S. R. (1976). Subpopulations of human T cells identified by receptors for immunoglobulins and mitogen responsiveness. *J. Immunol.* **117**, 2171.
Paul, W. E., and Benacerraf, B. (1977). Functional specificity of thymus dependent lymphocytes. *Science* **195**, 1293.
Shou, L. S., Schwartz, A., and Good, R. A. (1976). Suppressor cell activity after concanavalin A treatment of lymphocytes from normal donors. *J. Exp. Med.* **143**, 1100.
Shreffler, D., and David, C. S. (1975). The H-2 major histocompatibility complex in the immune region. *Adv. Immunol.* **20**, 125.
Stanton, T. H., and Boyse, E. A. (1977). A new serologically defined locus, Qa1, in the TL-A region of the mouse. *Immunogenetics* **3**, 525.
Strelkauskas, A. J., Schauf, V., Wilson, B. S., Chess, L., and Schlossman, S. F. (1978). Isolation and characterization of naturally occurring subclasses of human peripheral blood T cells with regulatory functions. *J. Immunol.* **120**, 1278.
Winchester, R. J., Fu, S., Wernet, P., Kunkel, H. G., Dupont, G., and Jersild, C. (1975). Recognition by pregnancy serums of non-HL-A alloantigens selectively expressed on B lymphocytes. *J. Exp. Med.* **141**, 924.

The Serology of HLA-A, -B, and -C

F. KISSMEYER-NIELSEN

Tissue-Typing Laboratory, University Hospital, Aarhus, Denmark

I. Introduction	99
II. Experimental Methods and Findings	100
III. Conclusions	109
References	111

I. Introduction

The HLA system is the human equivalent of the *H-2* system in the mouse, and knowledge about *H-2* has been of tremendous help in the exploration of the HLA system in man. The *H-2* system, as well as the HLA system, has been shown to constitute a very strong transplantation barrier, and both systems are determined by a very complex set of genes located on a single pair of chromosomes. The orientation of the loci belonging to the major histocompatibility complex of mice (*H-2*) and man (HLA) is depicted, somewhat simplified, in Fig. 1.

The *K* and *D* loci in mice are equivalent to the B and A loci, respectively, and the D or DR locus in man relates to the *I-A* complex in mice. The D locus determines the stimulation elicited in the mixed lymphocyte culture (MLC) in man, while the equivalent genes in mice are located in the *I-A* region. The *G* region in mice contains genes giving weaker MLC stimulation, and similar genes are most probably located in the neighborhood of the A locus in man. The products as

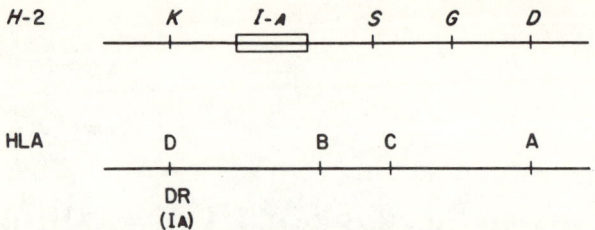

Fig. 1. The major histocompatibility system of mice (*H-2*) and of man (HLA).

coded for by the human A, B, C, and DR loci can be determined by serological techniques and were previously determined (SD, serologically defined). This is in contrast to LD determinants as coded for by the human D locus (LD, lymphocyte defined using the MLC reaction). It is still not known whether the DR locus is identical to the D locus or belongs to a separate locus closely linked to the D locus. It has been shown that the HLA genes are located on chromosome No. 6.

II. Experimental Methods and Findings

The HLA antigens seem to be present on the surface of all human cells, most of which could probably be used for typing. However, the concentration of HLA antigens on the surface varies from cell to cell, and lymphocytes (the total population of these cells, disregarding subpopulations) have been shown to be particularly suited for typing. The concentration of antigens is rather high, and these cells are rather easy to isolate using flotation on very well standardized gradients such as Ficoll–Isopaque (Lymphoprep), and utilizing small differences in specific gravity between erythrocytes, granulocytes, and lymphocytes—the lymphocytes having the lowest gravity. If defibrinated blood (often slight dilution in buffer) is layered on top of the gradient, which is subsequently centrifuged, erythrocytes and granulocytes go to the bottom and lymphocytes can be harvested from the interface and further processed for typing.

Cellular elements that can be used for typing are obtainable also from isolated platelets procured from stabilized blood by sedimentation and differential centrifugation procedures.

The basic principle in the two assay methods is similar. If an antiserum contains an HLA antibody active against an HLA antigen on the surface of living lymphocytes or stored platelets, complement present in the reaction mixture is fixed by the antigen–antibody complex. In the lymphocytotoxic technique, complement fixation induces holes in the cell membrane and viable lymphocytes are killed (= cytotoxicity). When platelets are used, the amount of complement fixed is measured by adding sensitized sheep red cells as in any complement fixation technique.

The principal steps in the lymphocytotoxic technique are summarized in Table I. The viable lymphocytes are usually procured from defibrinated peripheral blood, but excellent preparations may also be prepared from lymph nodes and spleens. The principal sources of antisera are also apparent from Table I, but it must be pointed out that it has been, and still is, extremely difficult to find good antisera reacting only with one HLA antigen (monospecific antisera). HLA antisera seem to have a marked tendency to be oligo- or multispecific, even when the phenotypes of donor and recipient imply exposure to only one antigen. This may be explained by the antisera becoming reactive with antigenic determinants, being shared by, or very similar in, several HLA antigens. This is an analogy to Rh serology, where immunization against the D antigen may result in production of antibodies active not only against red cells carrying the D antigen, but also against red cells that are C positive and D negative. Once again, this is most probably caused by the D and C antigens sharing the same antigenic determinants, called G. This is one of the main problems involved in HLA typing and histocompatibility testing at present.

The difficulties in finding large quantities of good antisera resulted in the development of a very elegant micromethod by Terasaki and

TABLE I
LYMPHOCYTOTOXIC MICROTECHNIQUE

Antigen	Isolated living lymphocytes
Antisera	Parous women
	Febrile transfusion reactions
	Immunization of volunteers with skin grafts, leukocytes, or platelets
Microtechnique in oil chambers	Antiserum, 1.0 µl; lymphocytes (2000–4000 cells) in 1.0 µl complement
	Visualization of killing of lymphocytes using various techniques—mostly staining of dead cells using trypan blue or eosin Y

McClelland in 1964. This microtechnique made it feasible to perform one test with less than 1 µl of antiserum and a few thousand isolated lymphocytes. All the cytotoxic techniques used today are modifications of Terasaki's original procedure. In the technique shown in Table I, a dye is used to visualize the cytotoxicity or killing, since this dye is taken up only by killed cells. Other possibilities for technical variations are available (see National Institutes of Health Manual for tissue typing).

A modified micromethod for the platelet complement fixation technique, which has recently been developed and has found wide application (Colombani *et al.*, 1971), is briefly outlined in Table II. These two techniques are most commonly used for HLA typing, especially in conjunction with histocompatibility testing. Each method has advantages and disadvantages; however, it should be stressed that the largest number of HLA antigens can be detected using lymphocytotoxicity, since it seems to be even more difficult to find antisera useful for the complement fixation assay than for the lymphocytotoxic technique.

Cross-reactivity between various HLA antigens has been a major problem in relation to the serological exploration of this very complex system. Cross-reactivity between antigens and antibodies is most probably caused by chemical (structural) similarities between the antigens involved. This results in a number of unexpected immunological features in relation to the HLA system.

1. Challenge with a single HLA antigen may result in production of

TABLE II
COMPLEMENT FIXATION TECHNIQUE WITH PLATELETS:
STANDARDIZED INTERNATIONAL MICROTECHNIQUE[a,d]

Component	Amount (µl)
Antibody (serum dilution or eluate)	2
Platelet suspension (500,000/µl)	2
Human complement diluted (2 H100 units in 2 µl)[b]	2
Sensitized sheep red blood cells (200,000/µl)[c]	2

[a] The test is performed in Falcon microtest tissue culture plates No. 3034 under mineral oil.

[b] Mix and incubate for 1 hour at 37°C.

[c] Mix and incubate for 30 minutes at 37°C; centrifuge and read on a serology reading box.

[d] For details see "Histocompatibility Testing, 1972."

an HLA antibody (antibodies) with a much broader reactivity than expected.

2. Absorption of an antiserum with a cross-reactive antigen may eliminate the antibody reactivity in spite of a negative antibody test, the so-called ANAP (agglutination negative absorption positive) or CYNAP (cytotoxicity negative absorption positive) phenomenon.

3. The cross-reactivity has also resulted in identification of antisera reacting with two or more cross-reactive antigens, which later were identified as separate entities when more "narrow" reagents became available. This has resulted in the so-called "splitting" of HLA antigens into increasingly "narrow" and rare antigens.

We would like to mention a few classical examples of this cross-reactivity and splitting of antigens: van Rood's *4a(= Bw4) specificity* has been shown to contain HLA-B5, B12 (= Bw44), B13, and some other rare B antigens. Similarly, van Rood's *4b (= Bw6) specificity* has been shown to contain B7, B40, Bw22, and a number of other specificities.

The picture of 4a and 4b as emerging from the seventh workshop in Oxford ("Histocompatibility testing, 1977") appears from Table III.

It should be stressed that it is impossible to find two 4a or two 4b antibodies having exactly the same reaction pattern. Nevertheless, they have been shown to be useful reagents in the definition of various splits, as appearing in Table III.

HLA-A28 was originally defined using an anti-HLA-A2, which also contained anti-HLA-A28; consequently A28 could be defined only in the absence of A2, which of course seriously hampered the exploration of this antigen.

HLA-A11 was similarly defined using duospecific antisera, which identified HLA-A3 + A11 until monospecific anti-HLA-A11 antisera were finally identified during the 1970 histocompatibility testing workshop.

The TT^x antigen (= Bw45) was for many years defined with some antisera containing anti-B12 (= Bw44) + anti TT^x (= Bw45), but very recently two monospecific anti-Bw45 sera have been described.

Another very typical example is the HLA-Aw19 antigen, which has been split into A29, Aw30, Aw31, Aw32, and Aw33.

The above-mentioned problems have caused some difficulties in precise HLA typing. If one does not have all the narrow monospecific reagents (which is very difficult to achieve), identity for one of the broader specificities may in fact imply incompatibility for one of the

TABLE III
Bw4 (4a) AND Bw6 (4b) AND THEIR RELATIONSHIP TO A AND B SPECIFICITIES[a]

Bw4		Bw6	
B5
Bw51
Bw52
Bw53		Bw35
B18	
Bw44
Bw49	B12
Bw21	Bw45
Bw50	
Bw"15.2"
B17	B15	Bw"15.1"	
Bw38	Bw16	Bw39	
B13
Bw47
B27		B40
Bw48
Bw41	
		B7
Bw42
Bw22	(w22.1)
(w22.2)
(Bw54)
		B14
B8	
B37			

[a] Horizontal lines separate clusters of cross-reactive specificities.

narrow specificities; this, of course, is very undesirable in the transplantation situation. However, in this situation the immunogenicity of the incompatible antigen seems to be rather low, and it has been difficult to demonstrate, for example, in kidney transplantation.

It might be reasonable to end this section relating to the HLA-A and -B series summarizing what is needed for laboratory work in this area in order to find and characterize new antisera. The following requirements are important:

1. To have experienced technicians.
2. To have a reliable and reproducible technique.

3. To have a highly selected and thoroughly HLA-typed panel of lymphocyte donors, which includes (if possible) all known HLA-A and -B antigens, and also known "blanks" (i.e., antigens for which no antisera are yet available).

4. To document that the postulated monospecific antiserum never reveals "triplets" (i.e., no person should have more than two antigens belonging to the antigenic series involved).

5. To do family studies in order to show that the antigen defined segregates as other antigens belonging to the same series, i.e. determined by a dominant genetic determinant, closely linked to the other "series" of determinants belonging to the HLA region.

The various points listed are not always easy to establish; some of them may not be completely reliable, and alternatives are available. The principal aim must be to find monospecific reagents; this may be achieved using the selected panel mentioned under point 3, but an alternative is the "statistical" approach testing against large random panels and calculating (using 2×2 tables) the χ^2 values for new sera against previously known antisera (or antigens). We are not very much in favor of this approach, as cross-reactivity may cause inclusions, and the well known linkage disequilibrium between various HLA antigens may easily result in high χ^2 values—without any real "identity" between the reagents involved.

The family studies should be able to confirm that the antigenic determinants investigated are encoded by genes of the "HLA region." However, this is definitely not a proof of the quality of the reagent investigated. Because of the extreme polymorphism of the HLA system, oligo- or even multispecific HLA antisera may perform nicely in families and show perfect agreement with expectations.

Point 4 above is very important and may be used to introduce the C series of HLA antigens (= third series or AJ series), which were originally proposed by the Scandinavian group during the Blood Transfusion Congress in Moscow in 1969 (see Thorsby et al., 1970).

The first antigen identified and proposed to belong to this new series of antigens was defined with a serum (AJ) originating from Lena Sandberg (Göteborg), and this antigen had a frequency ~4% in the Scandinavian population.

The criteria used for postulating that this antigen belonged to a new or third series of serologically defined antigens follow.

1. The antigen was found in many unrelated individuals possessing four well established HLA antigens, two A- and two B-series antigens.

2. There was no evidence for admixture of the AJ antibody component to other antisera as an explanation for the positive reactions (= triplets) obtained.

3. Absorption experiments supported the statements in the preceeding paragraphs.

4. Investigations of a large number of families show that the AJ gene "always" travels together with the same A and B genes. However, a few families with recombinations in the HLA region have shown "crossover" between the B and C loci, and other recombinations between A and B have shown that the sequence of the series on chromosome 6 must be A:C:B, or vice versa.

5. Capping experiments (not used originally, but introduced later).

Shortly after the original identification of the AJ antigen, it was found to be closely associated with the HLA antigens B5, Bw15, Bw22, and B27, and it was seriously considered that anti-AJ was a complex antiserum reacting with small but similar parts of the molecular structures of the previously mentioned B series of antigens. Thus the Aj antiserum could be another example of cross-reactivity within the same series of HLA antigens, and thus another example of falsely defined new loci as discussed by Kissmeyer-Nielsen and Thorsby (1970). However, during the sixth histocompatibility workshop ("Histocompatiblity Testing, 1975"), this third, or C series of antigens was more or less generally accepted. This was at least partly the result of elegant experiments performed by Solheim *et al.* and others. They used Fab_2 fragments of antibodies in blocking experiments and immunofluorescence with different markers for antibodies belonging to the individual HLA loci. The results of these experiments strongly indicate that the antigens of the C series belong to molecular structures, moving independently of the A and B antigens, and thus may be determined by a separate locus.

The experiments seem very convincing, but other explanations might be possible. The HLA antigens are known to be composed of several polypeptide chains, and we have speculated whether the antigen–antibody interaction might result in cleavage of some bonds between the polypeptide chains inside the HLA antigen molecules, thus giving a false impression of molecular independence of some antigenic determinants. This is purely speculative, but we have data that certainly do not favor the existence of a separate third series of serologically defined HLA antigens.

For a number of years we have been interested in the two-loci concept (A + B) of the serologically defined HLA antigens. In order to confirm or disprove this, we have selected a series of *strong, multispecific lymphocytotoxic antisera* originating from multitransfused and/or parous patients, where the antibody reacted with more than ~90% of our selected panel. The patients having the antibody were HLA typed, and subsequently we selected as many HLA-*identical* or -*compatible* individuals as possible from our still increasing panel of HLA-typed blood donors (by now more than 6000). We have considered in this respect also people differing from the antiserum donor only for one HLA antigen, which is supposed to cross-react with another HLA antigen possessed by the antiserum donor.

The results of our preliminary experiments were published several years ago, and it was concluded that the results strongly supported the two-loci HLA concept, i.e., the A and B loci. No evidence was found indicating a third locus. These experiments have been continued, and a summary of the results is shown in Table IV. The table includes the

TABLE IV

Multispecific Cytotoxic Antisera Tested against HLA-Identical and HLA-Compatible[a] Panel Donors, Considering Only A and B Antigens

Serum donor		HLA phenotype	Identical[b]		Compatible[b]	
			Neg.	Pos.	Neg.	Pos.
52664/72	G.M.	A2, 3; B7, 27	2	0	17	3
5524/71	D.H.	A3, 9; B7, 17	0	0	9	0
18543/71	C.C.	A1, 2; B7, 8	8	0	16	4
19651/71	A.M.	A1, 2; B7, 8	8	0	16	4
23780/71	N.H.	A1, 3; B7, 8	12	0	21	1
25471/71	K.A.	A3, w19; 12	1	0	6	0
27139/71	P.M.	A2, w19, B8, 40	0	0	4	0
5193/71	K.T.	A3, 11; Bw35, 7	3	0	0	0
43814/74	A.J.	A1, 11; Bw35, 8	5	0	6	0
57137/74	N.H.	A2, 28; B7, 40	0	0	9	0
15399/71	H.D.	A2; B12, 40	4	0	6	0
58737/72	A.B.	A3; B7, 18	0	0	6	0
11431/71	L.N.	A2; B15	3	0	0	0
23670/71	R.P.	A3; B7	5	0	0	1
59828/72	E.J.	A3; B7	5	0	0	1
			56	0	116	14

[a] Compatible = not full-house donors, but no identified incompatible antigen.
[b] Neg., negative; Pos., positive.

results obtained with multispecific antisera from 15 individuals. The most important finding is that no positive reactions were found among the 56 tests performed against A and B HLA-identical donors; in particular, there were no positives in the 39 full-house combinations. About 10% positives were found while testing against more than 100 compatible donors, but this might be explained by the presence of still undetectable antigens in the positive, not full-house (i.e., not all antigens defined), donors.

The experiments have been repeated using the same approach, but as we were at the same time looking for B cell-active antisera, we tested against enriched B cell suspensions in addition to normal lymphocytes. The experiment included 17 multispecific antisera tested in a chessboard pattern against lymphocytes from 31 selected panel donors. This included 10 HLA-A and -B identical combinations and 39 HLA-A and -B compatible situations. The results were very similar to those appearing in Table II. No positive reactions were seen in the 10 HLA-identical combinations; and in 3 out of the 39 compatible combinations, positive reactions were observed.

Unfortunately, only a minority of the serum donors were typed for the HLA-C specificities, but all the known C specificities were represented in the panel donors.

Once again the results of our experiments do not favor the existence of the C series of antigens, but it must be admitted that there are other explanations to our negative findings, including the two following ones.

1. The well-known and strong positive associations between the postulated C series of antigens and antigens belonging to the B series may explain our negative findings. If the associations between the HLA-B and C antigens are very strong, then most of the critical panel members could by chance possess the same C antigen as the HLA-identical, immunized serum donor. This would prevent antibody production against this particular C antigen. This is difficult to accept, however, as the number of experiments has increased.

2. Disparity for HLA-A and B antigens may be necessary, in some unknown way, for reactivity with the C series of antigens.

Further support for the two-loci HLA concept may rest on the following findings.

1. The HLA-A and B antigens have been found to influence kidney graft survival markedly, and there is no evidence at present as to a correlation between graft survival and C-series incompatibilities. How-

ever, there have been only a limited number of investigations in this respect.

2. The HLA-A and -B antigens have been shown to be very important targets in cell-mediated lympholysis (CML), and the influence of disparity for C series antigens is rather questionable.

3. In spite of intense, worldwide search for new HLA antisera, we can still only account for ~60% of the genes belonging to the C series.

4. Extensive immunizations of volunteers challenging against still unidentified C antigens have not been able to provoke anti-C antibodies. Consequently, these antigens must at least have a very low immunogenicity (Ferrara et al., 1977).

The above-mentioned recombinants between the A, C, and B series of genes are difficult to explain, but intragenic recombination is a possible explanation.

III. Conclusions

Our laboratory was involved in the original definition of the third (C) series of serologically defined HLA antigens. We have been following the arguments "pro et contra" ever since, and we have now accumulated data that argue against the existence of this series as a serological entity. We cannot disprove the existence of the C series, but we would like to warn against too firm acceptance and to wait for chemical analysis of the antigens to be done.

The picture of the HLA-A, -B, and -C antigens emerging after the workshop in Oxford ("Histocompatibility Testing, 1977") with the various antigens—including splits—appears in Table V.

It should be added that the antigens listed in Table V and the frequency of the corresponding genes, which can be easily calculated, account for 98–99% of the theoretically possible genes in most populations, when we consider the A and B series of antigens and genes. However, as previously mentioned, we still lack about 40% of the genes and antigens belonging to the C series, simply because of lack of the antisera necessary for their identification.

It should also be mentioned that the frequency of the various antigens and genes varies considerably from one ethnic group to another—and some genes seem to be virtually absent in some populations. This interesting aspect of the HLA system is not a part of the HLA-A, -B, and -C serology and will not be considered further, but it could be

TABLE V
Complete Listing of Recognized HLA-A, -B, and -C, Specificities[a,b]

New	Previous	New	Previous	New	Previous
HLA-A1	HL-A1	HLA-B5	HL-A5	HLA-Cw1	T1
HLA-A2	HL-A2	HLA-Bw51	5.1	HLA-Cw2	T2
HLA-A3	HL-A3	HLA-Bw52	5.2	HLA-Cw3	T3
HLA-A9	HL-A9	HLA-B7	HL-A7	HLA-Cw4	T4
HLA-Aw23	W23	HLA-B8	HL-A8	HLA-Cw5	T5
HLA-Aw24	W24	HLA-B12	HL-A12	HLA-Cw6	T7
HLA-A10	HL-A10	HLA-Bw44	B12, not TT^x		
HLA-A25	W25	HLA-Bw45	TT^x		
HLA-A26	W26	HLA-B13	HL-A13		
HLA-A11	HL-A11	HLA-B14	W14		
HLA-Aw19	Li	HLA-B15	W15		
HLA-A29		HLA-Bw16	W16		
HLA-Aw30		HLA-Bw38	W16.1		
HLA-Aw31		HLA-Bw39	W16.2		
HLA-Aw32		HLA-B17	W17		
HLA-Aw33		HLA-B18	W18		
HLA-A28	W28	HLA-Bw21	W21		
HLA-Aw34	Malay 2	HLA-Bw49	W21, SL		
HLA-Aw36	Mo^x	HLA-Bw50	W21^x		
HLA-Aw43	BK	HLA-Bw22	W22		
		HLA-Bw54	W22 (Japanese)		
		HLA-B27	W27		
		HLA-Bw35	W5		
		HLA-B37	TY		
		HLA-B40	W10		
		HLA-Bw41	Sabell		
		HLA-Bw42	MWA		
		HLA-Bw46	HS (Mongoloid)		
		HLA-Bw47	(407^x)		
		HLA-Bw48	(JA)		
		HLA-Bw53	HR		
		HLA-Bw4			
		HLA-Bw6			

[a] The "w" before the number indicates that the specificity is still not fully accepted.
[b] Splits of broader antigens are listed indented below the antigen in question; e.g., HLA-A9 with the two splits Aw23 and Aw24.

mentioned that the anthropological aspect of HLA was the main subject of the fifth workshop in histocompatibility testing held in Evian 1972 with Jean Dausset as chairman ("Histocompatibility Testing, 1972").

References

Ferrara, G. B., ed. (1977). "HLA System: New Aspects." Elsevier/North-Holland Biomedical Press, Amsterdam.
Götze, D., ed. (1977). "The Major Histocompatibility System in Man and Animals." Springer-Verlag, Berlin and New York.
"Histocompatibility Testing, 1965" (H. Balner, F. J. Cleton, and J. G. Eernisse, eds). Munksgaard, Copenhagen, 1965.
"Histocompatibility Testing, 1967" (E. S. Curtoni, P. L. Mattiuz, and R. M. Tosi, eds). Munksgaard, Copenhagen, 1967.
"Histocompatibility Testing, 1970" (P. I. Terasaki, ed). Munkşgaard, Copenhagen, 1970.
"Histocompatibility Testing, 1972" (J. Dausset and J. Colombani, eds). Munksgaard, Copenhagen, 1972.
"Histocompatibility Testing, 1975" (F. Kissmeyer-Nielsen,ed). Munksgaard, Copenhagen, 1975.
"Histocompatibility Testing, 1977" (W. F. Bodmer, J. R. Batchelor, H. Festenstein, J. Bodmer, and P. J. Morris, eds). Munksgaard, Copenhagen, 1977.
Kissmeyer-Nielsen, F., and Thorsby, E. (1970). *Transplant. Rev.* **4**.
Terasaki, P. I., and McClelland, J. D. (1964). Microdroplet assay of human serum cytotoxins. *Nature (London)* **204,** 998–1000.
Thorsby, E., Sandberg, L., Lindholm, A., and Kissmeyer-Nielsen, F. (1970). The HL-A system: Evidence of a third sub-locus. *Scand. J. Haemat.* **7,** 195–200.

The Serology of HLA-DR[1,2]

J. J. VAN ROOD and A. VAN LEEUWEN

Department of Immunohematology, University Medical Center, Leiden, The Netherlands, and Eurotransplant Foundation, Leiden, The Netherlands

I. Introduction 113
II. Technical Considerations 114
III. Results 118
IV. Discussion 120
    References 121

I. Introduction

The recognition of an immunogenetic system requires (as the name indicates) both an adequate immunological technique and reagents, and at least a basic understanding of the genetics of the system. It is obvious that these requirements can be the cause of formidable difficulties when it is attempted to recognize and describe a new system. The HLA-DR antigens are no exception.

---

[1] DR stands for D related. This indicates that, although the antigens that can be recognized by serology are related to the HLA-D determinants, it is by no means certain that they are identical to them.

[2] This work was supported in part by NIH contract NO2-A1-82553; the Dutch Foundation for Medical Research (FUNGO), which is subsidized by the Dutch Organization for the Advancement of Pure Research (ZWO); the Dutch Organization for Health Research (TNO); and the J. A. Cohen Institute for Radiopathology and Radiation Protection (IRS).

Although the recognition of the HLA-A and -B antigens could be systematically worked out since 1962, when an appropriate method was published, it took another 10 years and partly new methodology to attain the same for HLA-DR. This was not only because it took several years before it was recognized that the determinants that stimulated in mixed lymphocyte culture (MLC) were not identical to HLA-A and -B (as originally assumed), but also because it took even longer before it was accepted that the HLA-D locus was polymorphic, like the HLA-A and -B loci, and methods to recognize this polymorphism became available. As a matter of fact, the analysis of HLA-D and -DR took place simultaneously.

Much of the pressure to search for methods to type for HLA-D and especially DR came from those involved in clinical organ transplantation. It had already been recognized that low or negative MLC reactivity improved graft survival of both skin and kidneys in man and of kidneys also in monkeys. It was clear that one way of selecting MLC-negative (or weak reacting) donor–recipient pairs for kidney transplantation when postmortem donors had to be used was to be able to type them for HLA-D, i.e., the system responsible for the strongest stimulation in the MLC test. Although typing with homozygous typing cells and the primed L-determinant typing (PLT) test provided that service as outlined in this volume by Bach and Sondel, the methods were considered by many to be more time consuming and costly and less reliable than a serological method, if such a method could be developed. In fact, there existed considerable scepticism that this would be feasible. Much of this scepticism was based on the fact that in many other systems T cell-dependent immunity differed in its specificity and antigenic requirements from B cell-dependent immunity.

II. Technical Considerations

That we decided to study the problem of HLA-D related serology was in no small way due to observations by Ceppellini and his co-workers (1971), who had in a large study confirmed and extended observations of others showing that sera with anti HLA-A and -B antibodies were able to inhibit the MLC test. Although MLC inhibition by HLA antibodies was thus a well established phenomenon, the mechanism by which this occurred was (and to a large extent still is) poorly understood. When we decided to use the MLC inhibition technique to screen for anti HLA-DR antibodies, it was clear from the beginning that the test system had to be rigorously controlled to be certain that irrelevant antibodies (i.e., other than anti HLA-DR) could not cause MLC inhibition. To attain this, we used responder cells for the MLC that were obtained from the person—in most cases a woman with a history of multiple pregnancies—who had formed the leukocyte antibodies. If MLC inhibition occurred we could be assured that this was in all probability due to an antibody reacting with the stimulator lymphocytes. To exclude interference by anti HLA-A and -B antibodies, stimulator cells were used that were HLA-A and -B identical to the responder cells. We have named this approach the MLC inhibition test using SD identical stimulator cells, MISIS for short. The sera that were tested contained strong anti HLA-A and/or -B antibodies. This was done on the assumption that persons who were able to produce strong anti HLA-A and/or -B antibodies might likewise also be able to produce anti HLA-DR antibodies. The very first serum tested in the MISIS test was informative (Table I). Some responder–stimulator cell combinations (P, N, T, U, V, W) were inhibited whereas others (Q, R, S) were not. This finding was reproducible, and other sera showing similar results were found easily.

TABLE I
Typing for HLA-DR: Mixed Lymphocyte Culture (MLC) Inhibition and Immunofluorescence[a]

	AB serum (cpm)	Serum Sch (cpm)	AB serum/ serum Sch[b]	Fluorescent (% positive cells)
Sch + P_m	3,300	400	7.3	17
Q_m	14,000	8000	1.7	4
N_m	9,700	1100	9.5	17
R_m	10,000	6400	1.6	9
S_m	4,200	2800	1.7	7
T_m	5,200	700	7.4	7
U_m	13,500	1300	10.0	16
V_m	26,500	1100	24.1	17
W_m	1,800	200	10.0	—

[a] All stimulator cells were SD identical with the responder cells of parous woman HLA-A2, A3, B7, Bw40.

[b] Inhibition index values obtained by dividing the counts per minute obtained by culturing the cells in AB serum by the counts per minute obtained when they were cultured in serum Sch. The significant inhibitions are italicized (van Leeuwen et al., 1973).

Next we asked the question whether MLC inhibition was really due to an antibody. This seemed likely because the MLC inhibiting activity could be absorbed by stimulator cells that were inhibited. More direct evidence that antibody mediated MLC inhibition was obtained when van Leeuwen together with Schuit developed a sandwich immunofluorescence test with anti-IgG which, for these days, gave an unusually low background with normal lymphocytes. Whereas in the background staining 4–8% of the cells fluoresced, some of the stimulator cells when tested with the serum used in the MISIS test showed bright staining of 16–17% of the cells (Table I). The low background immunofluorescence was clearly essential to detect these small differences and was originally dependent on very rare and very pure rabbit anti human Ig sera (courtesy of J. Ràdl, Laboratory of Experimental Gerontology, Rijswijk). When it was understood that the background staining was due to binding of fluorescein-labeled immunoglobulins by Fc receptor molecules, commercially available sera were subjected to pepsin treatment to remove the Fc part of the anti human Ig and the test became generally available.

As is illustrated in Table I, the first serum to detect polymorphism in the MISIS test showed also significant positive fluorescence. The results of the two tests correlated quite well, a finding that was substantiated in latter studies. The MLC-inhibiting substance remained stable for years. On the basis of this and other considerations, it was assumed that the MLC-inhibiting substance and the antibody that reacted in the immunofluorescence test were probably the same, and thus an IgG molecule.

The next question that had to be resolved was why only such a small percentage of the cells of peripheral blood reacted with these antibodies. This turned out to be due to the fact that these antibodies reacted with a determinant present on B cells and monocytes but absent from (most) T cells and platelets. The latter observation had practical consequences because it provided a simple means of purifying the anti-DR reagents: platelets lack DR but carry HLA-A, -B, and -C antigens and are thus ideally suited to remove anti HLA-A, -B, and -C antibodies from serum, while retaining the anti HLA-DR antibodies.

When this information became available it was logical to test the antibodies found in the MISIS and/or immunofluorescence tests by complement-dependent cytotoxicity. Early attempts failed because in man the number of B cells in peripheral blood is low. But when B cell-enriched cell suspensions became available through depletion of T cells by rosetting with sheep red blood cells, this problem was easily overcome, and it could be shown that many of the sera contained complement-dependent cytotoxic antibodies that reacted with B cells and monocytes. Prolonged incubation times further increased the efficacy of the long B cell or rosetting technique. The test was standardized and used during the seventh histocompatibility workshop ("Histocompatibility Testing 1977").

Although the rosetting B cell test is quite adequate when investigating healthy individuals, B cell enrichment methods are tedious and, with the blood of patients suffering from some diseases, quite difficult.

To circumvent this obstacle a further refinement was introduced. Instead of enriching the B cells in the test cell suspension, they were identified with fluorescein-labeled sheep anti human Ig. The monocytes stain as well. Next a standard two-stage complement-dependent lymphocytotoxicity test was carried out, and the dead cells were identified by means of ethidium bromide. The red fluorescence of the latter stain and the green of the first can be read simultaneously by appropriate selection of (blocking) filters.

With this, the two requirements for the detection of the HLA-DR antigens had been fulfilled: adequate techniques and reasonably pure antibodies were available (Table II).

The genetics of the system did not offer too much of a problem either, because it was assumed from the beginning that HLA-D and -DR were, if not identical, very closely related to each other. While the techniques were developed for HLA-DR typing as described above, the study of HLA-D using homozygous typing cells had progressed quite rapidly (see review by Bach and Sondel in this volume). Our group was especially fortunate because Keuning, Termijtelen, and co-workers had typed a large-sized panel and a number of families for HLA-D with homozygous typing cells, which enormously facilitated the comparison of the distribution of HLA-D versus HLA-DR. The results showed that

TABLE II
DEVELOPMENT OF HLA-DR SEROLOGY

1. Identify sera that possibly contain anti HLA-DR by a modified mixed lymphocyte culture inhibition test (MISIS)
2. A low background anti-Ig immunofluorescence test detects that anti HLA-DR antibodies react with B cells but not with T cells
3. B cell-enriched suspension and platelet-absorbed sera make it possible to use the complement-dependent cytotoxicity test for the detection of HLA-DR

in the Dutch Caucasian population the distribution of HLA-D and -DR was very similar. Herewith the next prerequisite of basic understanding of the genetics appeared to be resolved as well.

III. Results

Figure 1 depicts the distribution of HLA-DR as compared to HLA-D. There is striking similarity between D and DR, especially for the determinants 1, 2, 3, and 7. Agreement for 4, 5, 6 and 8 is, although highly significant, less good. This could be due to unavailability of optimal antibodies when this study was done, but other explanations can not be ruled out (see below).

Inspection of Fig. 1 shows that the number of triplicates, i.e., individuals carrying three (instead of the expected two) DR determinants is quite small and could easily be explained by assuming that the sera used contained antibodies against more than one determinant. The Hardy–Weinberg fit is good, and family studies are also compatible with the assumption that the HLA-DRw1–7 and wIA8 are codominant alleles of one locus; if they are not identical to the HLA-D determinants, they are very closely linked to them. The data collected during the seventh histocompatibility workshop confirmed and extended these findings. The sum of the gene frequencies of HLA-DRw1 to 8 is near one. If these determinants are indeed coded for by one locus, then these findings taken together would imply that most of the DR determinants have already been identified.

It is by no means certain, however, that this simple concept will turn out to be correct. Sasportes, Dausset, and co-workers (1977) have presented preliminary evidence that HLA-D as recognized by homozygous typing cells is not identical to HLA-DR, but that the structures recognized by the PLT test are. Other investigators, including our own group, have more recently made observations that could be compatible with the above assumption.

Also the concept that D or DR determinants, or both, are alleles of one locus might be an oversimplification. Although the number of triplets is small in Dutch Caucasians, it might be larger in individuals from India. More extensive studies, preferably with anti HLA-DR antibodies found in the population where the study is done, are needed to settle this point. One could summarize the present position by saying that the information available so far is still compatible with the assumption that one locus codes for most of the DR determinants, but

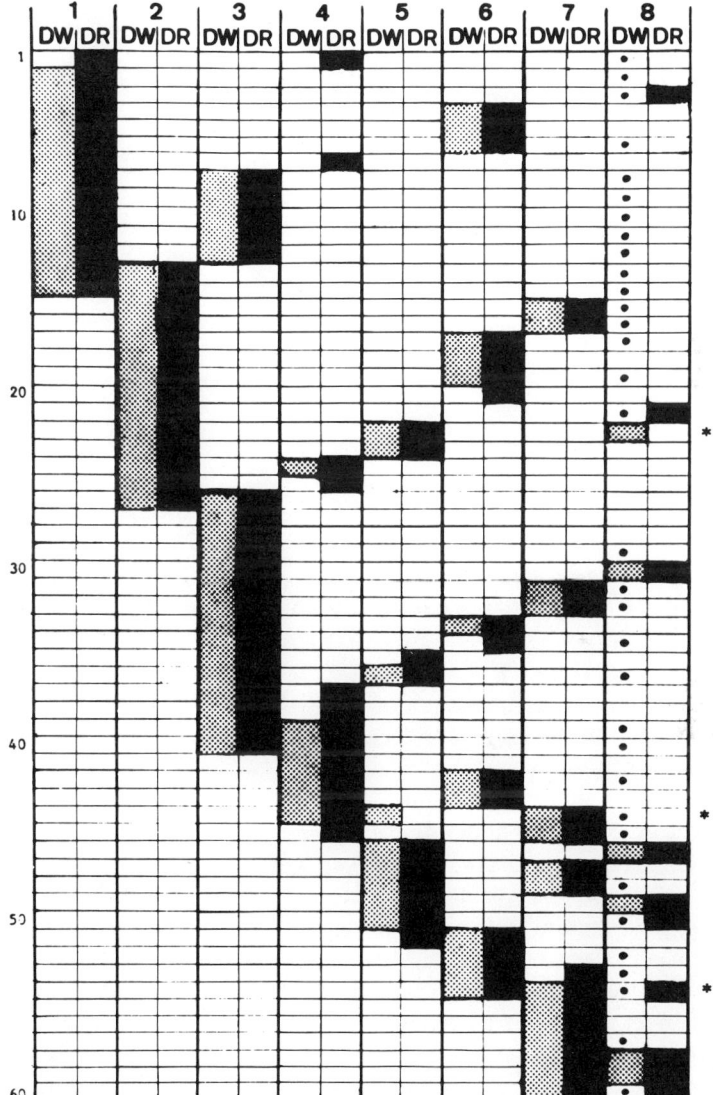

Fig. 1. Lymphocytes of 60 unrelated donors were tested by HTC and PLT recognizing the HLA-D specificities HLA-Dw1-8. The positive results are indicated by ▓. The same panel was tested in by sera recognizing HLA-DRw1-7 and HLA-wIA8 (positive results, ■). Note the excellent agreement of the results obtained with cellular (HTC and PLT) and serological (HLA-DR serology) techniques for the determinants 1, 2, 3, and 7. The number of possible triplets is only one for HLA-DR, suggesting that HLA-DR determinants might be coded for one locus. ●, Not done; *, possibility of triplets not formally excluded.

that, although these determinants are at least very closely linked to the HLA-D determinants, it is by no means certain that the two are identical. There are some first indications that "splits" exist of the DR determinants.

A few reports indicate that determinants present mainly on B cells are coded for by loci other than the HLA-DR locus. Some of them are probably located in HLA, other appear to be coded for loci outside HLA. The recognition and description of the determinants is still in its infancy.

IV. Discussion

This chapter set out to describe the serology of HLA-DR and to give some information on the genetics of HLA-DR as well. We have presented the data more or less in the chronological order in which they were collected. Needless to say, the tradition of generous exchange of reagents and information that is so typical for the HLA field was of enormous help in the analysis of this fascinating set of genetic markers.

In this context the work of Walford and his collaborators should be mentioned, because they identified anti HLA-DR antibodies using a completely different approach. Walford originally wanted to study antigens present on leukemic cells only. He choose for this the cells of chronic lymphoblastic leukemia (CLL) patients and showed that such leukemic cells carried antigens that appeared to be absent from normal cells. Only much later it became clear that the CLL cells, which as a rule are B cells, carried DR antigens, just as do B cells from healthy donors, and what at first appeared to be a system of "leukemic" antigens was in fact at least in part the DR antigen series. Walford called these antigens the Merrit system. He has recently published evidence that the Merritt system might consist of two series of multiple alleles.

About the techniques used by us to detect the HLA-DR antibodies, we can be brief. The concept of MISIS was crucial. The principle of the method, i.e., use of target cells that are HLA identical with the donor of the antibody producer can be used for the analysis of all minor histocompatibility systems. It has recently been applied successfully to the detection of monocyte antibodies, which appear to be important in bone marrow rejection.

For the analysis of the specificity of the HLA-DR antibodies, panels typed for HLA-D by homozygous typing cells were used. In this manner, it was relatively easy to identify sera with antibody specificities that were virtually identical to those recognized by homozygous typing cells. This procedure is highly efficient but it carries the risk of bias; in other words, sera with antibodies that do not correlate well with the HLA-D specificities stand a good chance of not being analyzed further. For this reason, it is reassuring that an unbiased 2×2 analysis carried out during the seventh histocompatibility workshop came up with precisely the same results. The sera discussed here are thus the most frequent B cell antibodies. As we already mentioned, it is well possible that B cells carry fewer immunogenic determinants coded for by loci other than the HLA-DR locus.

Clinical urgency in organ transplantation provided an important stimulus for the development of HLA-DR serology. The first results correlating DR matching with graft survivial have come in and look extremely promising (see discussion by van Rood and Persijn in this volume). Also for disease association studies, the tool of DR serology will be of paramount importance, especially for the study of those diseases for which predisposing genes are not in close linkage disequilibrium with the HLA-A, -B, or -C antigens, e.g., in rheumatoid arthritis and tuberculoid leprosy.

In the long run one of the most important consequences of HLA-DR serology might well be that it enables us to study the chemistry of yet another cell surface structure, a structure that might be involved in self and non-self recognition.

References

Bach, F. H., and van Rood, J. J. (1976). *N. Engl. J. Med.* **295**, 806, 872, 927.
Ceppellini, R., Miggiano, V. C., Curtoni, E. S., and Pellegrino, M. A. (1971). *Transplant. Proc.* **III**, 63.
Claas, F. H. J., van Rood, J. J., Warren, R. P., Storb, R., and Su, P. J. (1979). *Transplant. Proc.* **XI**, 423.
"Histocompatibility Testing 1977" (W. F. Bodmer, J. R. Batchelor, H. Festenstein, J. Bodmer, and P. J. Morris, eds.). Munksgaard, Copenhagen, 1977.
Legrand, L., and Dausset, J. (1975). *Transplant. Proc.* **VII**, 5.
Mann, D. L., Albelson, L., Harris, S., and Amos, D. B. (1976). *Nature (London)* **259**, 145.
Sasportes, M., Fradelizi, D., Nunez-Roldan, A., Giannopoulos, Z., and Dausset, J. (1977). *Tissue Antigens* **10**, 162.

van Leeuwen, A., Schuit, H. R. E., and van Rood, J. J. (1973). *Transplant. Proc.* **V**, 1539.
van Leeuwen, A., Winchester, R., and van Rood, J. J. (1975). Ann. N. Y. Acad. Sci. **254**, 289.
van Rood, J. J., and van Leeuwen, A. (1963). *J. Clin. Invest.* **42**, 1382.
van Rood, J. J., van Leeuwen, A., Keuning, J. J., and Blussé van Oud Alblas, A. (1975). *Tissue Antigens* **5**, 73.
van Rood, J. J., van Leeuwen, A., and Ploem, J. S. (1976). *Nature (London)* **262**, 795.
van Rood, J. J., van Leeuwen, A., Persijn, G. G., Lansbergen, Q., Goulmy, E., Termijtelen, A., and Bradley, B. A. (1977). *Transplant. Proc.* **IX**, 459.
Walford, R. L., Gossett, T., Troup, G. M., Gatti, R. A., Mittal, K. K., Robins, A., Ferrara, G. B., and Zeller, E. (1976). *J. Immunol.* **116**, 1704.
Walford, R. L., Ferrara, G. B., Gatti, R. A., Leibold, W., Thompson, J. S., Mercuriali, F., Gossett, T., and Naeim, F. (1977). *Scand. J. Immunol.* **6**, 393.

Cellular Immunogenetics—Definition of HLA-D Region Encoded Antigens by T Lymphocyte Reactivities[1]

FRITZ H. BACH and PAUL M. SONDEL[2]

Immunobiology Research Center and Department of Medical Genetics, University of Wisconsin, Madison, Wisconsin

I. Introduction	124
II. Mixed Leukocyte Culture with Homozygous Typing Cells	127
A. Methods	127
B. Homozygous Typing Cells	127
C. Results	128
III. Primed LD-Typing (PLT)	132
A. Methods	132
B. Results	134
C. Pool-PLT	138
D. Discussion	140
IV. General Discussion	141
References	142

[1] This work is suppored in part by NIH grants AI 11576, AI 08439, CA 16836 and National Foundation grants 1-246 and 6-78. This is paper No. 187 from the Immunobiology Research Center and paper No. 2343 from the Laboratory of Medical Genetics, The University of Wisconsin, Madison, Wisconsin.

[2] Present address: Department of Pediatrics, CSC, 600 Highland Avenue, Madison, Wisconsin 53706.

I. Introduction

Specific cell surface antigens or antigenic determinants have been classically defined by serological methods, which with respect to HLA have been reviewed elsewhere in this volume. An alternative approach is to utilize the reactivity of T lymphocytes to "define" antigens based on the belief that the determinant(s) that are recognized by T lymphocytes may not be identical to those recognized by antibodies. It is for this reason that parallel and complementing terminologies have been used to reflect this difference.

In man, the currently defined antigens of the HLA system have been separated into two types of antigens by both genetic mapping and functional tests. A working terminology that allows separation both of the two "types" of loci as well as the two methods for the detection of determinants associated with those loci is shown in Table I. Other

TABLE I
TERMINOLOGY FOR SEROLOGICALLY AND T CELL-DETECTED ALLOANTIGENS[a]

Method	HLA	
	D	ABC
Serology	DR	SD
T cell responses	LD	CD

[a] Differential terminologies for the antigens detected by serological methods and by studying T cell responses are used on the assumption that the determinants recognized by the two methodological approaches are not identical. The determinants recognized as serologically related to the D locus are referred to as the DR (D-related) antigens; those recognized as products of the HLA-A, -B, and -C loci, as the classical SD (S determinant) antigens. The antigens recognized with T cell responses are the LD (L determinant) antigens. These are the antigens that stimulate most of the proliferative response in a primary mixed leukocyte culture; it is not clear, as discussed in the text, whether they are identical to the antigens that stimulate a primed LD type of (PLT) response. The LD antigens as defined with homozygous typing cells are the products of the HLA-D locus. The CD (C determinant) antigens recognized by cytotoxic T lymphocytes are associated with the HLA-A, -B, and -C loci.

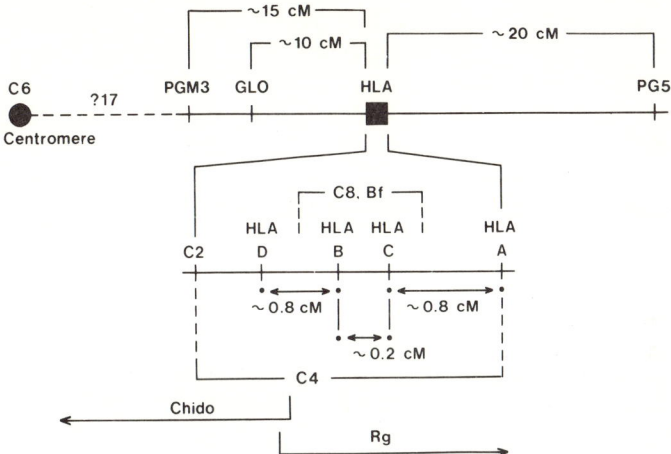

Fig. 1. Schematic representation of the HLA region on the sixth chromosome. In the top part of the figure is given the map of chromosome C6. The phosphoglucomutase-3 (PGM3) locus is approximately 17 centimorgans (cM) distant from the centromere, on the basis of data on ovarian teratomas. That locus, as well as glyoxylase (GLO) and urinary pepsinogen-5 (PG5), is given, with the respective distances from HLA. The HLA complex is represented in an enlarged version in the lower part of the figure. The HLA-A, -B, -C, and -D loci are shown as well as their distances from each other in centimorgans. In addition, the location of the locus for complement-factor 2 (C2) is given. The locus for complement-factor 4 (C4) is between the locus for C2 and HLA-A; the loci for complement-factor 8 (C8) and properdin-factor B (Bf) are located in the region indicated—their exact localization has not yet been ascertained. Similar localization for the Chido blood group and the Rogers (RG) blood group are indicated so far as knowledge is now available.

chapters in this volume describe the detection of the HLA-A, -B, and -C controlled antigens both by specific antisera and by cytotoxic T lymphocytes. Our purpose in this article is to review the cellular methods that are available for detection of antigens associated with the HLA-D locus. We shall refer to the HLA-D region as that segment of chromosome 6 that has been separated from HLA-B by recombination and includes the HLA-D locus as defined in a primary mixed leukocyte culture (MLC). A schematic representation of the HLA chromosome as our knowledge has evolved is shown in Fig. 1. The reason for referring to an HLA-D "region" as well as the HLA-D locus is the following. The HLA-D locus was defined using a primary MLC; the specific antigens of that locus were defined by using homozygous typing cells (as reviewed below) in a primary MLC. In a formal sense, any other antigenic determinant(s) related to HLA-D but detected by another method could be present either on a different part of the molecule encoded for by the HLA-D locus or on a molecule encoded by genes that are very closely linked to HLA-D but not identical to HLA-D. It is for this reason that the "serologically defined" antigens that are genetically mapped to the HLA-D region are referred to as DR, or D-related, rather than assuming them to be identical to the HLA-D antigens defined by homozygous typing cells in MLC. We must therefore caution that antigens of the HLA-D region detected by cellular methods other than homozygous typing cells, including the primed L determinant (LD) typing (PLT) test (see below), may or may not be measuring products of the HLA-D locus itself.

The HLA-D locus was established as being separate from the HLA -A, -B, and -C loci based on findings in many families showing that non-HLA antigens do not stimulate in MLC and on family studies in which cells of siblings who were identical for the HLA-A, -B, and -C antigens stimulated each other very strongly in a primary MLC test. Other MLC combinations within those families demonstrated that by far the most lymphocyte stimulation was due to antigens controlled by a locus linked to but distinct from the HLA-A, -B, and -C loci; that locus is now known as HLA-D. Prior studies have shown that all stimulation in MLC using healthy cell donors whose cells had not been sensitized *in vivo* is due to the HLA complex itself. Thus the HLA-D antigen(s) is functionally defined as that antigen which stimulates primary MLC responses. The magnitude of stimulation in primary MLC as it is usually performed, provides meaningful quantitation of the degree of HLA-D disparity. It does not, however, allow specific identification (i.e., typing) of the HLA-D antigens. What is needed are "reagents" similar to the anti HLA-A, -B, and -C sera that specifically type for the HLA-D antigens. The difficulty is that these antigens are recognized by cells rather than by sera.

We shall discuss here three separate cellular "typing" systems used to identify antigens of the HLA-D region. The following will be discussed: first, the use of homozygous typing cells in the primary MLC; second, the use of primed LD typing; and third, the use of pool-priming in an attempt to obtain a cellular "cross-match" assay of the incompatibility strength between two individuals as it relates to these tests.

II. Mixed Leukocyte Culture with Homozygous Typing Cells

A. METHODS

For the most part, MLC methods that are now used involve microtechniques in which cells are cultured in the wells of microtiter plates, each well holding 0.1–0.2 ml and a total of between 25,000 and 100,000 responding cells. Cells used both as responding and stimulating cells in an MLC are purified from peripheral blood by separation on a Ficoll–Hypaque gradient in which the red blood cells and granulocytes sediment through the Ficoll–Hypaque gradient whereas the lymphocytes and monocytes are retained at the interface. These cells are recovered from the interface and washed in tissue culture medium with human plasma or serum. "Responding" cells are used directly after washing; "stimulating" cells are pretreated either with X-irradiation or mitomycin C. Both of these agents prevent the stimulating cells from incorporating radioactive thymidine into DNA and yet still allow them to present their cell surface antigens to the responding cells in a stimulatory manner.

The MLC is assayed by adding radioactive thymidine, $[^3H]TdR$ on day 4 or 5 of the culture and measuring the radioactivity incorporated into the cells of each culture after 6–12 hours of exposure to the $[^3H]TdR$. Even though MLC responses are detected on days 6, 7, or 8, it is best to quantitate the response magnitude when the stimulation is still showing a continuing and steady increase. Obviously, inaccurate quantitative data, in terms of any comparison, will be obtained if one MLC is already on a plateau value of response on a given day of assay whereas another MLC is still increasing very markedly. Comparisons should thus be made on a day when all the cultures to be compared are still in a growth phase where no inhibitory conditions are yet detected.

B. HOMOZYGOUS TYPING CELLS

The use of homozygous typing cells are introduced by Mempel, Grosse-Wilde, and their collaborators and is based on one of Sir Peter Medawar's "laws" of histocompatibility. He demonstrated that two separate, highly inbred (homozygous) strains, let us call them AA and

BB, would readily reject skin grafts from one another. However, an (AB)F$_1$ animal from these two strains was unable to recognize either parent as foreign, and no skin rejection would result. Similarly, cells of individuals heterozygous for their HLA-D antigens are unable to respond to stimulating cells that are homozygous for either of those HLA-D antigens.

The basis of using homozygous cells for HLA-D *typing* is the following. First, one must collect lymphocytes from several individuals homozygous for HLA-D. Each homozygous individual is assigned a distinct HLA-D antigen specificity. Those individuals whose lymphocytes do not stimulate each other are assigned the same specificity. To then "type" any given unrelated individual, the lymphocytes of that individual are stimulated in separate MLCs with stimulating cells from each distinct homozygous typing cell (HTC). If cells of that individual do not show a significant response against a given HTC then it is presumed that the cells of that individual carry the HLA-D antigen(s) of that HTC. If cells of a given unrelated individual do respond significantly to an HTC, then those responding cells presumably do not carry HLA-D antigen(s) of the HTC. The theoretical basis of assigning an HLA-D antigen, thus, is that the responding cell will not show reactivity to an HTC carrying that antigen (see Table II).

Two types of HTCs can be used. The first comprises cells that are *genotypically* homozygous in that there is a common ancestor and the two HLA chromosomes carried by that individual are presumably identical in descent since they both come from that common ancestor. Alternatively, two individuals can be considered *phenotypically* homozygous on the basis that their cells behave as HTCs both within families and in an unrelated panel.

Family testing should demonstrate that HTCs from a sibling do not stimulate responding cells of any member in that family who carries one haplotype identical with the haplotypes of the HTC. In unrelated panel studies, a given HTC should show a discriminatory response pattern in a panel in that the HTC either does not stimulate responding cells of some unrelated individuals or stimulates those cells significantly less than it stimulates responding cells of others.

C. RESULTS

Testing the responding cells of a number of unrelated individuals with a given HTC used as a stimulator can give any one of a number

TABLE II
ASSIGNMENT OF HLA-D ANTIGENS USING HOMOZYGOUS TYPING CELLS (HTCs)[a]

Responder	Stimulating HTC	[^{3}H]TdR incorporated (cpm)
A	(A$_x$)	328
A	DW1	1,063
A	DW2	28,411
A	DW3	1,944
A	DW4	38,662
B	(B$_x$)	119
B	DW1	18,012
B	DW2	24,837
B	DW3	21,008
B	DW4	33,592

[a] Results with only one HTC for each of the "antigens" DW1 through DW4 are given. These results allow the assignments of antigens DW1 and DW3 to individual A; individual B appears to have none of the four antigens for which HTCs were included in the experiment.

of different "patterns" of response. Some HTCs will, in most cases, yield highly discriminatory results in that the cells of some responders will respond very little to that HTC, whereas cells of all other individuals will respond very strongly. The "biphasic" nature of such a response allows the division of individuals tested into two groups: first, those that give a low or zero response to the HTC; second, those that give a significantly greater response. Individuals in the first group are then said to carry the HLA-D "antigen" of that HTC.

A pattern such as that just described is rarely found when considering all the different HTCs used for HLA-D typing. Much more frequently the responses of different individuals to the HTC vary from very low values, in terms of counts per minute of [^{3}H]TdR incorporated, to very high values. Sometimes such distributions can be divided by statistical analysis into two separate distributions that are not readily apparent by simply looking at the data. Several different methods have been suggested to perform such analyses; these methods will not be discussed here but can be found in the reviews and books referenced at the end of this chapter. All the methods are aimed to establish the "level" of "relative response" (as discussed later in this article) below which a "typing response" can be said to have taken place. A typing response is equated with the presence of the HLA-D antigen on the responding cells that is present on the HTC.

The concept of a "relative response" has had important influence on interpreting HLA-D typing with HTCs. The question being asked in HTC typing is whether a given responding cell shows an abnormally low response to the HTC consistent with "identity" for HLA-D. Obviously, the counts per minute of [^{3}H]TdR incorporated will depend in part on the "responsiveness" of the tested individual's responding cells. Thus, included in every experiment are positive control stimulating cells; some laboratories use a mixture of many individuals' lymphocytes as their positive control, others take the average stimulation by three separate random individuals as their control. In any case the object is to provide an MLC stimulus that should induce a significant MLC response in all individuals tested; this response can then be considered to be a "100% response." The response in counts per minute of particular responding cell to each HTC can then be compared to the response shown by cells of that individual to these control stimulating cells and can thus be expressed as a percentage "relative response" when compared to the 100% positive control response. This approach represents "normalization" of the response with respect to the responding cell.

Some laboratories using HTCs for HLA-D typing will accept relative responses as high as 40% as still being consistent with a typing response, whereas others require a relative response less than or equal to 25%. However, equating such a "typing response" with HLA-D identity is probably a simplification of what is probably the basic immunogenetic situation. For instance, several different HTCs, obtained from different unrelated individuals, can be used to help "define" a given HLA-D antigen. Yet, those different HTCs will, in many cases, stimulate each other to quite a significant degree in a primary MLC test, suggesting lack of complete identity for HLA-D. In addition, it has been demonstrated that typing responses using different HTCs can show "inclusion" phenomena. That is, individuals who give a typing response to one HTC may all give a typing response to a second HTC, although there may be individuals who give a typing response to the second HTC who do not give a typing response to the first HTC. These findings suggest that a "typing response" in this system identifies individuals whose HLA-D antigens are immunologically similar, but not necessarily identical to those on the HTC. One again should recall the absence of MLC response when individuals are known to be HLA-D identical by pedigree analysis as with HLA identical siblings.

Thus two HTCs, presumably defining the *same* HLA-D antigen, may actually define two very similar yet distinct antigens. Such findings argue for complexity of the HLA-D region and are consistent with the hypothesis that an individual who gives a typing response to a given HTC, or even several different HTCs used to define a given HLA-D antigen, may not carry exactly the same HLA-D determinants expressed on any one of the HTCs used in that study. In other words, it appears (as is discussed in sections to follow) that a single HLA-D haplotype can code for several different HLA-D determinants; a typing response might thus indicate that one of the responder haplotypes shares most, but not all of the HLA-D determinants expressed by the HTC. Only the total lack of response would suggest identity for all determinants.

Even with the above reservations, the HTC method has been used internationally to identify and standardize HLA-D antigens as defined by this technique. Note that unrelated individuals who are HLA-D identical by this kind of typing often stimulate one another quite strongly in MLC. Nevertheless, the information provided has been invaluable in population genetic studies, identifying disease associations and predicting magnitude of MLC responses and even graft rejection.

TABLE III
CURRENTLY RECOGNIZED DW "ANTIGENS"[a]

Antigen	Gene frequency in Caucasoids	Most significant HLA-B association[b]
DW1	7.4	Bw35, (B27)
DW2	10.6	B7
DW3	9.2	Bi, (B18)
DW4	5.2	(Bw44), (B15)
DW5	7.6	B14, (Bw51)
DW6	10.2	(Bw22)
DW7	7.8	B12, B13, B17
DW8	2.1	—
DW9	—	—
DW10	—	—
DW11	11.0	B17

[a] Taken from "Histocompatibility Testing 1977," p. 362.
[b] Parentheses around antigen designations indicate less significant associations.

Listed in Table III are the presently defined HLA-DW antigens together with gene frequencies and the most common association with the HLA-B antigens as defined serologically. It is to be expected that each of these antigens will in the future be "split" into several different antigenic determinants and that there may be sharing of determinants between what are now considered to be different DW antigens as just discussed.

III. Primed LD-Typing (PLT)

The PLT test was devised to provide a more rapid assessment of D region encoded antigens. At the present time, as already suggested above, it is not clear whether the determinants recognized by PLT cells are identical with those that stimulate in a primary MLC. We shall thus refer to the HLA-D region-controlled antigens that are detected by the PLT method as PL determinants until their relationship to HLA-D has been further clarified.

A. Methods

The PLT test was based on the observation that cells that are stimulated in MLC and allowed to revert to small nonprolifering cells several days beyond the peak of the proliferative response have been "primed" to the sensitizing antigens on the stimulating cells in the primary MLC. If such primed cells are now "restimulated" with cells carrying the same antigens present on the stimulating cells in the primary MLC, a very rapid proliferative and cytotoxic response will develop against those antigens. The response of the primed cells is frequently referred to as a "secondary-type" response. It was the observation from our own laboratory that the secondary proliferative response was primarily engendered by antigens of the HLA-D region that led to the concept of primed LD typing for D region antigens.

Lymphocytes of one individual are stimulated in a primary MLC (usually in a flask to accommodate more cells) with mitomycin C or X-irradiated stimulating cells differing from the responding cell donor by one known haplotype (i.e., in parent–child combinations or by stimulating with homozygous typing cells). In either case the immunogenetic disparity presented to the responding cells in the primary MLC (the "sensitizing" MLC) is minimized as compared with the admixture of cells of unrelated cells that in most cases will differ by two HLA-D haplotypes. In contrast to the primary MLC, which requires 3–4 days to detect significant [^{3}H]TdR incorporation, the "secondary" response can be detected by [^{3}H]TdR uptake as early as 24 hours after "restimulation." X-irradiated or mitomycin C-treated cells from the responding cell donor provide no recognizable foreign HLA-D antigen, and thus restimulation with these gives a value for "control," background proliferative activity. Restimulation with cells of any other individual would give varying results depending on whether that other individual carries the PL antigens to which the cells were sensitized in the initial MLC. We refer to the restimulating cells that come from the same individual who was the donor of the sensitizing cells for the primary MLC as the "reference cell"; to the control restimulating cells as "control" cells; and to restimulating cells from any third-party individual as "test" restimulating cells.

To study the PL determinants in a population, multiple primary MLC combinations using many unrelated responding cell donors were each stimulated with different stimulating cells differing from the responder for a single haplotype. The secondary lymphocytes collected from each primary culture are then labeled "PLT cells" and are each stimulated in secondary cultures with a panel of unrelated stimulating cell donors. "Discriminatory" PLT cells are then selected; these are PLT cells that yield high proliferative responses when confronted with either the reference or some test cells, presumably carrying the PL antigens measured by that particular PLT cell, and give very low responses to restimulating cells that presumably do not carry those antigens. Using a discriminatory PLT cell, one can readily discern which restimulating cells carry the HLA-D region encoded determinant measured by that PLT cell and which do not. The PLT cells that do not provide this broad discrimination can still be analyzed in some cases by computer programs designed to test which restimulating cells can be statistically separated from others in terms of yielding a positive or a negative response (similar to the approach used with HTCs). Some PLT cells are relatively nondiscriminatory. Shown in Fig. 2 are results testing three different PLT cells against a panel of approximately 50 restimulating cells.

It is not yet understood why PLT cells fall into these different categories with regard to their ability to discriminate; although technical problems are one possible explanation, it is also possible that most

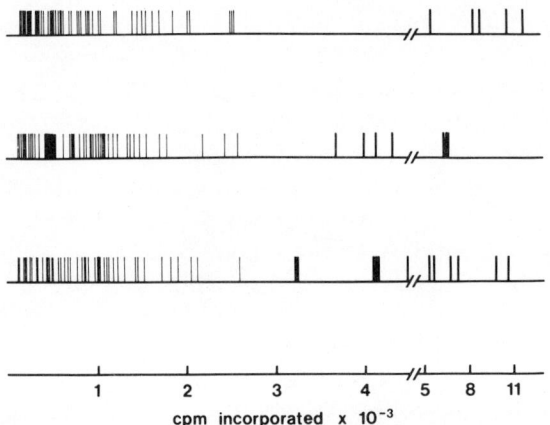

Fig. 2. Each vertical bar represents the response obtained with a given restimulating cell. Each primed L-determinant typing (PLT) cell was restimulated with approximately 50 different, unrelated restimulating cells. The first of three discriminatory PLT cells can be easily utilized to pick out the five individuals who give a strong response and thus carry the antigen(s) measured by that PLT cell. The second PLT cell can be used similarly, although with a somewhat lesser degree of confidence, to pick out the seven highest stimulating individuals. The third PLT cell is more difficult to analyze, especially with respect to the two individuals who restimulate on the order of 32,000 cpm.

nondiscriminatory PLT cells have been primed to many different PL determinants and the restimulating cells tested fall into many different groups in terms of the number of the determinants that they share with the original sensitizing cells of the primary MLC. Under these circumstances one would expect that some restimulating cells would restimulate a great deal and one might have all gradations of restimulation below that down to the control level.

In order to measure the many different PL determinants associated with HLA-D, a number of different PLT cells must be prepared so that reagents (PLT cells) would be available to measure all the existing PL determinants.

B. RESULTS

Shown in Table IV are results using PLT cells that were prepared within a family and restimulated on day 10 with cells from each family member. The PLT cell in this case was primed to the c haplotype in the family, and it is clear that only cells of those individuals in the family who carry the c haplotype restimulate to a significant degree.

Shown in Fig. 3 are results of testing a random panel with many different PLT cells. A number of different PLT cells are available for each of the PL specificities, as they have been referred to, in this figure. Thus, the first eight individuals listed on the left all seem to carry a determinant referred to as PL1 in the sense that cells of these individuals cause high restimulation of PLT cells $7BC_x$, $CBSA_x$ and $11BC_x$. Similarly, individuals 1, 7, 42, 43, 6, and 47 seem to carry an antigen referred to as PL2 since cells of these individuals restimulate the two PLT cells $9CB_x$ and $5CB_x$. In all, seven different PL antigens are defined by the studies presented in this figure. Interestingly, one antigen,

TABLE IV
24-HOUR PRIMED L-DETERMINANT TYPING

Individual haplotype	c
F = ab	239
M = cd	1863
C_1 = ac	1963
C_2 = bc	1807(S)[c]
C_3 = ad	281
C_4 = bd	−8
C_5 = bd	0(R)[c]
C_6 = bd	39
Background	364

[a] Used with kind permission of authors and publishers from Sheehy et al. in "Histocompatibility Testing 1975," pp. 414–458. 1975.

[b] Two PLT cells were prepared within a family. The father (F) was arbitrarily assigned haplotypes a and b and the mother (M) haplotypes c and d. The segregation of the parental haplotypes to the children (C) was determined by doing HLA S determinant (SD) typing. The PLT cell was prepared by stimulating the cells of child 5 with the cells of child 2. Since these two children shared the b haplotype inherited from the father, the cells of child 5 can recognize only the c haplotype on the cells of child 2. This PLT cell responds maximally only when restimulated with cells carrying the c haplotype.

[c] Responder and stimulator for primary culture used to prepare PLT cell.

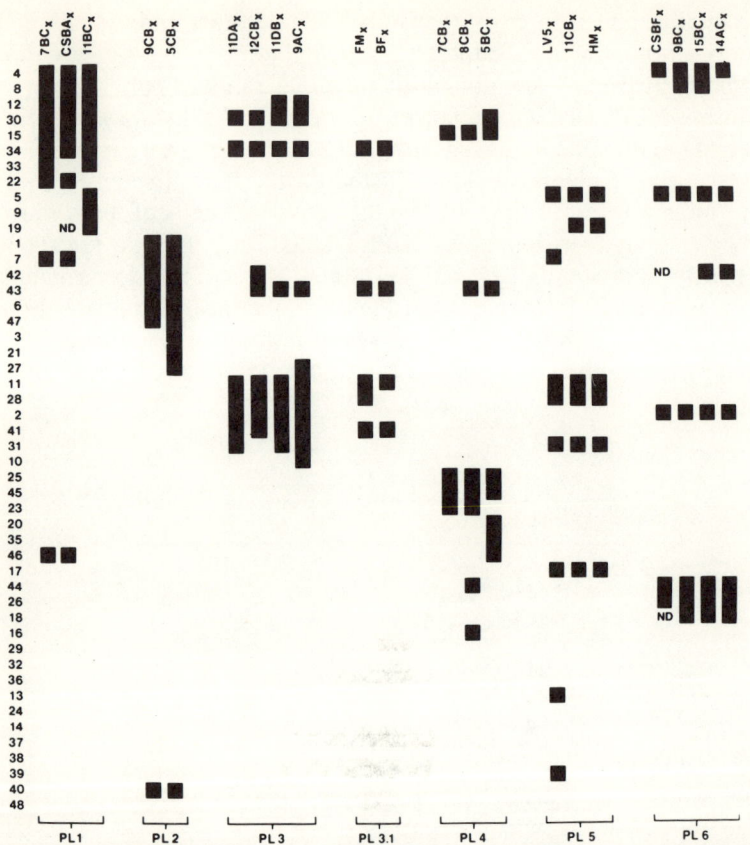

Fig. 3. Twenty-one different primed L determinant (LD) typing (PLT) cells listed across the top of the figure were tested against a panel of 48 unrelated test cells. The vertical black bars indicate those combinations of test restimulating cells and PLT cells that gave positive restimulation.

PL3.1 is "included" in PL3. That is, all individuals who bear PL3.1 also express PL3, although some individuals who are PL3 positive are PL3.1 negative. There is evidence, discussed in the original publication of these data, suggesting that even a single HLA-D haplotype codes for more than one PL determinant, paralleling the results with HTCs and attesting to the complexity of the D region.

The PL antigens are closely related to antigens that are defined with homozygous typing cells as well as to the determinants recognized by

CELLULAR TYPING OF HLA-D ENCODED ANTIGENS

anti-DR sera. In Fig. 4, PLT cells prepared against single haplotypes in family combinations are restimulated with a random panel that have been typed for their DW antigens. Very clearly there is an association between certain PL and DW antigens as, for instance, PL2 and DW2, PL5, and DW1. This association does not necessarily imply identity,

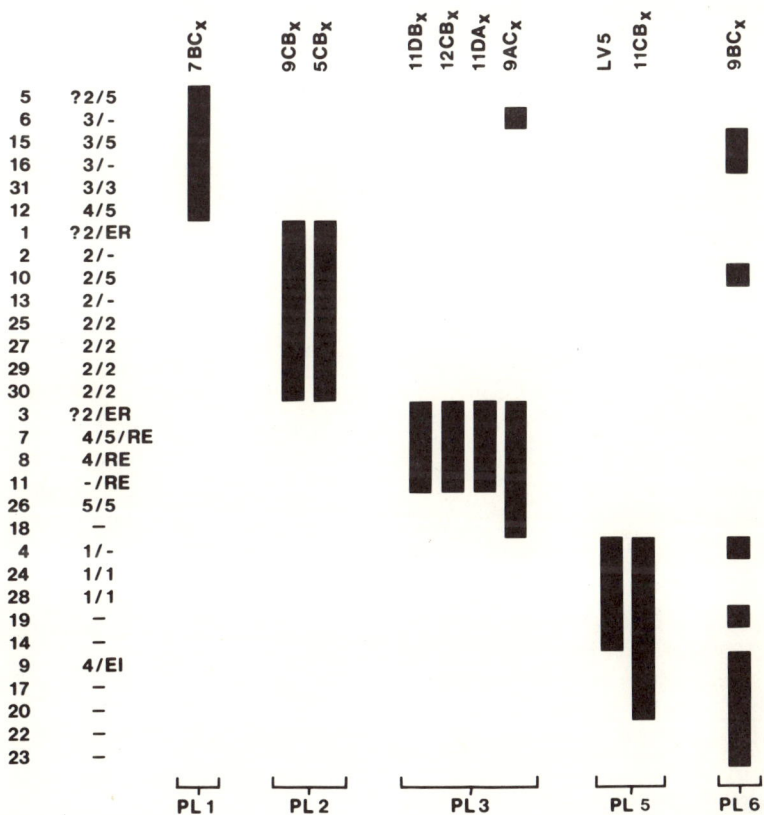

Fig. 4. The 10 different primed L determinant (LD) typing (PLT) cells listed across the top of the figure were tested against a panel of 30 unrelated test cells. Numbers listed on the left refer to the specific restimulating cell and its DW haplotype. Restimulating cells 17 and 18 gave no typing response. Cells 14, 19, and 20 have not yet been homozygous typing cell (HTC) typed, nor have cells 22 and 23, which in family mixed lymphocyte culture studies appear to be HLA-D homozygous. The vertical black bars indicate those combinations of test restimulating cells and PLT cells that gave positive restimulation. The numbers given at the bottom are the PL antigen designations assigned to these PLT cells in Madison before their use with the Tübingen restimulating panel.

since the determinants could be encoded by very closely linked genes that for the most part are found together on any single haplotype (a phenomenon referred to as linkage disequilibrium).

From such studies one finds evidence for the association, but also further evidence for complexity. Presented in Table V are actual data of restimulation of four PLT cells, defining two different PL determinants, by four different HTCs. In these selected and limited data, it is clear that PL3 is associated with DW6, a finding for which far more extensive data exist. However, in addition, it would appear that PLT cells measuring PL1 are restimulated not only by HTCs for DW3, but also by the homozygous typing cell for DW6. Thus, whereas there is an association between PL1 and DW3, there may also be an association between PL1 and DW6. One means to reconcile this apparent dichotomy would be to postulate that PLT cells for PL1 recognize a determinant that DW3 and DW6 share, but do not detect the determinants for which DW3 and DW6 differ.

Similar data exist from a number of different laboratories indicating an association between PL and DR, as defined serologically. In fact, associations exist in all combinations, as might be expected between the DW antigens defined with HTCs, the PL antigens defined with PLT cells, and the DR antigens defined serologically. As mentioned earlier, the precise relationship or possible identity between the HLA-D region antigens, DW, DR, and PL, awaits further clarification, and we must therefore continue to study these potentially separate antigens by all three methods.

C. Pool-PLT

The pool-PLT test was initiated as an attempt to provide a rapid "cross-match" for the amount of HLA-D disparity between two individuals. This would, it is hoped, be a rapid cellular assay that correlates with the primary MLC, which has been shown previously to be a biologically meaningful, quantitative measure of the amount of HLA-D disparity. The rapidity of the test might allow its use in human cadaveric transplantation, where organ preservation is still limited to 48–72 hours.

The pool-PLT utilizes a stimulating pool of mitomycin C- or X-ray-treated lymphocytes from 20 unrelated individuals in the sensitizing phase. We have previously shown that such a pool will stimulate a

TABLE V
RESTIMULATION OF PRIMED L DETERMINANT CELLS WITH HOMOZYGOUS TYPING CELLS

Restimulating cell	PD1		PL3	
	7BC$_x$	11BC$_x$	11DB$_x$	9AC$_x$
DW1	774	499	951	138
DW3	3509	2181	841	1030
DW3	6431	4833	213	1580
DW6	3232	4331	3299	7948

maximal proliferative response from any immunocompetent individual in a primary MLC. By sensitizing an individual's lymphocytes to this pool, PLT cells are produced that should give a secondary response to each PL determinant expressed on all of the 20 pool members. If the pool thus expresses the bulk of PL determinants in the population, the second response stimulated by any test individual will reflect the degree of recognizable PL antigens shared by the stimulator and the pool; that is, the greater the identity for PL antigens between the responder and test stimulator, the fewer the number of foreign, recognizable PL determinants on the stimulator. Thus the pool-PLT should correlate directly with primary MLC results. Table VI demonstrates that this is the case.

A pool-PLT cell was prepared with cells of individual A as the responding cells of the primary sensitizing MLC. Cells of individual A

TABLE VI
POOL-PLT CELLS: CORRELATION OF PRIMARY (1°) AND SECONDARY (2°) RESPONSES[a]

48-hour pool PLT		5-day 1° MLC	
Cells	[^{3}H]TdR (cpm)	Cells	[^{3}H]TdR (cpm)
AP$_x$ + A$_x$	477	AA$_x$	641
+ B$_x$	1,613	AB$_x$	2,527
+ C$_x$	14,128	AC$_x$	13,411
+ D$_c$	16,505	AD$_x$	23,068
+ HP$_x$	19,529	A(HP)$_x$	20,005

[a] HP stands for human pool, used as a standard both in terms of restimulation of the pool primed L determinant typing cells (PLT) and the primary mixed leukocyte culture (MLC).

were sensitized to the pool and then restimulated not only with cells of individual A, but also with cells of a number of unrelated individuals. Low restimulation of the pPLT cell by restimulating cells of an unrelated individual could be attributed to at least one of two phenomena. First, the D region PL antigens carried by the cells of that individual may not be represented in the pool, and thus the cells of that individual do not restimulate significantly. Second, the PL antigens on the restimulating cells may be shared in large measure with the PL antigens of the responding cell donor, and thus priming to those antigens was not possible. One can discriminate between these two possibilities on the basis of primary MLC data given in Table VI. The very close correlation between low restimulation of the pool-PLT cell and low stimulation of the primary MLC provide data supporting the concept that the pool-PLT is predictive of primary MLC and is a meaningful measure of the amount D region disparity between responder and pool-PLT restimulator.

D. Discussion

The PLT test was devised as an attempt to provide a rapid method of defining the D region antigens present on the cells of any given individual. In the great majority of cases strong restimulation of a PLT cell is caused by determinants encoded in the D region. Clearly a number of different PL antigens can be measured by generating a large number of PLT cells in one haplotype different family combinations. One of the great advantages of the PLT test is that reagents can be readily prepared in combinations where the stimulating cells carry determinants for which no homozygous typing cell or anti-DR serum is currently available. To the extent that PL determinants are different from DW or DRW, the PLT test provides complementary information about the immunogenetics of the HLA-D region.

As mentioned earlier, evidence exists from several lines of investigation suggesting that the D region is complex in terms of the number of determinants encoded by single D haplotypes. Since PLT cells can be readily prepared in any particular combination, it is to be anticipated that reagents will become available that would help to dissect this region. Since PLT results can be obtained after only 24 hours of culture, this test may become applicable for donor–recipient pairing, even prospectively, using cadaver kidneys.

An approach, already under investigation in some centers, is to use the pool-PLT test prospectively. This test allows one to sensitize cells of all potential recipients awaiting renal transplantation to the pool, freeze the pool-PLT cells, and then, when a cadaver donor becomes available, test which of the pool-PLT cells indicates the best HLA-D region match between that particular donor and a potential recipient. The potential advantage of using a cellular test such as the pool-PLT test for donor–recipient pairing over typing for the DR antigens serologically is that the pool-PLT test should provide biologically meaningful, quantitative data. Data regarding DR antigen matching might then be used in conjunction with the cellular response data from pool-PLT to hopefully predict optimal graft matching.

IV. General Discussion

We have attempted to review in this chapter the various methods that are currently used for examining the HLA-D region. The primary MLC test provides a biologically meaningful and quantitative measure of the amount of HLA-D disparity between two individuals, although the influence of determinants encoded by genes outside the HLA-D region on the level of response has been documented and must be considered in evaluating such results. The use of homozygous typing cells in a primary MLC has provided highly useful data regarding the polymorphism for the HLA-D region and has provided evidence suggesting that HLA-D region is complex, as discussed in various sections of this chapter.

Strong responses evoked in PLT cells are related primarily, if not solely, to the HLA-D region. This then provides yet another method of investigating the determinants associated with this gene complex. Rather than using unprimed, naive responding T lymphocytes, the responding cells in the PLT assay are cells that have already been primed *in vitro*. It is not clear whether the PL determinants recognized by PLT cells are identical with those recognized in a primary MLC.

One would have to conclude at the present time that the HLA-D region is complex certainly in regard to the number of different determinants encoded by genes in that region, including the HLA-D locus or loci. To which extent the HTC and PLT methods measure the same determinants or overlapping sets of determinants, and how these cellularly defined determinants are related to the determinants recognized by the anti-DRW sera (discussed in this volume by van Rood and van Leeuwen), will have to remain a topic for further investigation.

The importance of the HLA-D region in providing meaningful prognostic data for kidney allograft survival was first documented utilizing MLC tests and later anti-DRW typing (as reviewed in this volume by van Rood and van Leeuwen). In order to understand which determinants encoded within the D region are important in this regard, it will be necessary to understand the "strength" of the various determinants with regard to the cellular responses that they evoke leading to graft rejection and the probable relationship of the strength of the determinants to the genotype of the recipient.

References

Bach, F. H., and Hirschhorn, K. (1964). Lymphocyte interaction: a potential histocompatibility test in vitro. *Science* **143**, 813–814.

Bach, F. H., and van Rood, J. J. (1976). The major histocompatibility complex—genetics and biology. *N. Engl. J. Med.* **295**, 806–813, 872–878, 927–936.

Bain, B., Vas, M. R., and Lowenstein, L. (1964). The development of large immature mononuclear cells in mixed leukocyte cultures. *Blood* **23**, 108–116.

Dupont, B., Hansen, J. A., and Yunis, E. J. (1976). Human mixed lymphocyte culture reaction: genetics, specificity, and biological implications. *Adv. Immunol.* **23**, 107–202.

"Histocompatibility Testing 1975" (F. Kissmeyer-Nielsen, ed.). Munksgaard, Copenhagen, 1975.

"Histocompatibility Testing 1977" (W. F. Bodmer, J. R. Batchelor, J. G. Bodmer, H. Festenstein, and D. J. Morris, eds.). Munksgaard, Copenhagen, 1977.

Mempel, W., Grosse-Wilde, H., Baumann, P., Netzel, B., Steinbauer-Rosenthal, I., Scholz, S., Bertrams, J., and Albert, E. D. (1973). Population genetics of the MLC response: Typing for MLC determinants using homozygous and heterozygous reference cells. *Transplant. Proc.* **V**, 1529–1534.

Sheehy, M. J., Sondel, P. M., Bach, M. L., Wank, R., and Bach, F. H. (1975). HL-A LD (lymphocyte defined) typing: A rapid assay with primed lymphocytes. *Science* **188**, 1308–1310.

Sondel, P. M., Sheehy, M. J., Bach, M. D., and Bach, F. H. (1975). The secondary stimulation test (SST): A rapid LD matching technique. "Histcompatibility Testing 1975" (F. Kissmeyer-Nielsen, ed.), pp. 569–575. Munksgaard, Copenhagen.

Cell-Mediated Lympholysis[1]

DOLORES J. SCHENDEL

*Institute for Immunology, University of Munich,
Munich, Federal Republic of Germany*

I.	Introduction	143
II.	Terminology	145
III.	Technique	146
IV.	Specificity of Cell-Mediated Lympholysis	147
V.	Genetic Control of CML	148
VI.	Cell-Mediated Lympholysis Typing	151
	A. Procurement of Cytotoxic Typing Lymphocytes	153
	B. Standardized Target Cell Panels	154
	C. Definition of Positive and Negative Responses	154
	D. Analysis of the Specificity of Cytotoxic Lymphocytes	155
	E. Selection of Cells Identical for New Target Specificities	156
VII.	Preliminary Information from CML Typing Experiments	157
VIII.	Future Prospects	158
	Suggested Reading List	160

I. Introduction

The immunological response leading to rejection of a foreign tissue graft is very complex. Lymphocytes of the immune system recognize

---

[1] This work was supported in part by NIH grants CA-17404, CA-22507, CA-19267, CA-08748, and EY-01616.

foreign histocompatibility antigens and are stimulated to divide and infiltrate the graft. Some lymphocytes are activated to secrete various biologically active molecules, including specific antibodies that may enhance the rejection process. Other lymphocytes become cytotoxic and are capable of causing specific damage to the foreign tissue cells.

Three characteristics demonstrate the immunological basis of this cytotoxic response. One, the cells that mediate the destructive activity are thymus-derived lymphocytes (T cells). Two, they display an immunological memory, responding in an accelerated and enhanced manner when they are reexposed to the same foreign antigens to which they were initially sensitized. Three, the cytotoxic response they mediate is specific.

Cytotoxic lymphocytes have been identified *in vivo* during rejection periods following transplantation of foreign tissues and *in vitro* following stimulation with foreign lymphocytes in the mixed lymphocyte culture (MLC). The test system used to measure the destructive function of cytotoxic lymphocytes is called the cell-mediated lympholysis (CML) assay.

Although cytotoxic lymphocytes obtained after *in vivo* sensitization have been tested directly in CML, the most extensive studies of cell-mediated cytotoxicity have used the indirect *in vitro* MLC–CML technique. When lymphocytes from individual A are cultured with inactivated (X-irradiated or mitomycin C-treated) lymphocytes from individual B, they recognize foreign antigens expressed by B. This initial recognition results in enlargement and division of the A-responding lymphocytes and is designated as the MLC response. After incubation for 5–6 days in MLC, some A cells acquire the ability to lyse B cells, and this destructive function is measured in CML. The CML assay consists of incubating cytotoxic lymphocytes with radioactively labeled target cells. Direct cell-to-cell contact of cytotoxic lymphocytes with target cells results in membrane damage to the target cells, and subsequent osmotic changes cause target cell death and release of radioactive label into the surrounding medium. Measurement of the amount of radioactivity in the culture medium can then be used to quantify the degree of cytotoxicity directed against a target cell population. Initially, studies of cytotoxicity using the *in vitro* CML assay were restricted by the limited availability of suitable cell lines for use as target cells. Cell-mediated lympholysis analysis is now generally applicable because peripheral blood lymphocytes can be used as target cells.

II. Terminology

Cell-mediated lympholysis (CML) is the term used to designate the destructive function that cytotoxic *cells mediate* against *lymphocyte* target cells. This cytotoxic activity is independent of antibody and complement. Cytotoxic lymphocytes sensitized *in vivo,* for example, through transfusion or transplantation, are used in the *direct* CML assay, whereas cytotoxic lymphocytes sensitized *in vitro* are used in the *indirect* CML assay.

The cells causing lysis of target cells are called *cytotoxic lymphocytes* or *effector* cells. Their activity in CML is tested with three types of target cells. Cells identical to the responding cells in the MLC are called *autologous control* target cells, cells identical to the MLC stimulating cells are called *specific* target cells; and cells obtained from other unrelated individuals are called *third-party* target cells.

Lymphocytes from one individual are activated to become cytotoxic when they are exposed to *allogeneic* cells, that is, cells obtained from an individual of different genetic origin. The allogeneic stimulating or sensitizing antigens for cytotoxic lymphocytes are controlled primarily by the *HLA region.* Within this region antigens determined by the *HLA-A, -B, or -C loci* may be recognized by cytotoxic lymphocytes. Definition of these antigens is discussed in this volume by Kissmeyer-Nielsen.

HLA-D or -DRw antigens may also be involved in CML. Definition and characterization of these antigens is presented in this volume by van Rood and van Leeuwen and Bach and Sondel.

Other antigens determined by the HLA region are identified with the CML assay. These are presently referred to as *new target determinants* until more precise definitions can be made. Antigens controlled by genes that are not linked to the HLA region are called *non-HLA determinants.*

Every individual receives from each of his parents one chromosome that determines an HLA region. The genetic unit inherited from each parent is called an *HLA haplotype,* therefore a child inherits one maternal HLA haplotype and one paternal HLA haplotype. Occasionally, an exchange of genetic material occurs between two HLA haplotypes, resulting in a *recombinant HLA haplotype,* which is passed on to a child. An HLA haplotype contains a set of genes controlling the HLA-A, -B, -C, -D, and -DRw antigens, as well as other new antigens. It has been observed in population studies that some combinations of antigens of a single HLA haplotype occur more frequently than would be expected on the basis of their individual frequencies. This phenomenon is called *linkage disequilibrium*.

III. Technique

A schematic representation of the MLC–CML technique is shown in Fig. 1. The assay is performed in two stages. In the first step, cytotoxic lymphocytes are sensitized in a 6-day MLC, and in the second step their cytotoxic activity is measured in the CML assay. Peripheral blood lymphocytes from two allogeneic individuals, A and B, are separated from heparinized whole blood on density gradients. The stimulating cells from B are given 2000 rads of X-irradiation to block their ability to proliferate. Cells from A are cocultured in MLC with B_x stimulating cells in a tissue culture flask containing culture medium supplemented with human serum. The flask is incubated for 6 days at 37°C in an atmosphere of 5% CO_2. During this time, some of the A cells become sensitized to the alloantigens of B. On day 6 these sensitized cells are examined for their cytotoxic activity in CML. Preparation of the target cells is initiated 48–72 hours before the CML assay. Lymphocytes from individual B are isolated from peripheral blood and usually stimulated with the plant lectin phytohemagglutinin (PHA). Stimulation with PHA causes the lymphocytes to enlarge into blast cells, which are very sensitive to lysis by specific cytotoxic lymphocytes. On the day of the CML assay these target cells are incubated with radioactive sodium chromate, $Na_2^{51}CrO_4$, which is taken into their cytoplasm.

The AB_x cytotoxic lymphocytes are mixed with ^{51}Cr-labeled B target

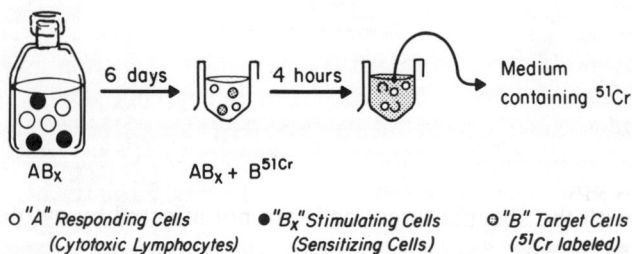

Fig. 1. The indirect mixed lymphocyte culture–cell-mediated lympholysis technique.

cells in small test tubes or individual wells of a microtiter plate and allowed to interact, normally for 4 hours. During this time cytotoxic lymphocytes are able to damage the target cells, resulting in the release of ^{51}Cr label into the culture medium. Thereafter the supernatant medium is removed and its content of ^{51}Cr label is determined. Two control cultures must be included in each CML test: spontaneous release of ^{51}Cr label from the target cells is determined either by incubating target cells with AA_x cells, which do not mediate any cytotoxicity, or by incubating target cells in medium alone; maximum release of ^{51}Cr label is determined by directly physically damaging the target cells by repeated freezing and thawing or exposure to detergent.

The experimental ^{51}Cr release caused by cytotoxic lymphocytes is expressed as a percentage of the maximum ^{51}Cr release caused by direct physical damage of the target cells, after correction for spontaneous release. The formula for the calculation is as follows:

$$\% \text{ CML} = \frac{\text{experimental release} - \text{spontaneous release}}{\text{maximum release} - \text{spontaneous release}} \times 100.$$

The percentage of CML increases when greater numbers of cytotoxic lymphocytes are incubated with a constant number of target cells. This allows quantitative comparison of the strength of CML responses by cytotoxic lymphocytes obtained from different MLC combinations.

IV. Specificity of Cell-Mediated Lympholysis

It is well established that CML displays specificity both at the level of induction of cytotoxic lymphocytes in MLC and at the level of target cell destruction. For example, responding cells cultured in MLC with autologous cells do not develop cytotoxic potential, but the same responding cells sensitized to allogeneic cells develop into specific cytotoxic lymphocytes. These cytotoxic lymphocytes cause little or no damage to autologous control target cells, whereas they cause extensive damage to specific target cells. These allosensitized cytotoxic lymphocytes can also lyse third-party target cells if they share determinants with the specific target cells. Third-party target cells not sharing antigens with the specific target cells are not affected by cytotoxic lymphocytes.

The specificity of target cell destruction is clearly demonstrated in "innocent bystander" experiments. If cytotoxic cells are incubated with radioactively labeled autologous control target cells and unlabeled specific target cells, no significant release of radioactivity is detected, thus the innocent bystander, or autologous control, target cells are not damaged. Inhibition experiments in which unlabeled target cells are added to a mixture of cytotoxic lymphocytes and labeled target cells also confirm this specificity. Under appropriate conditions, a linear decrease in the release of radioactivity from labeled specific target cells is observed with the addition of greater numbers of identical unlabeled specific target cells. Alternatively, addition of an excess of irrelevant unlabeled third-party target cells has little effect on the release of radioactivity.

The high degree of specificity expressed by cytotoxic lymphocytes implies that these cells have receptors specific for determinants on the surface of target cells. The strongest evidence supporting this concept comes from monolayer adsorption analysis. If AB_x cytotoxic lymphocytes are incubated on a monocyte or fibroblast monolayer of B cells, cytotoxic lymphocytes attach to this monolayer and can destroy the cells of the monolayer. The nonadsorbed cells mediate little CML damage to a second B monolayer, but if the adsorbed cells are eluted from the B monolayer, they are more potent in their ability to damage B target cells. This increased CML activity is probably due to an enrichment in the number of specific cytotoxic cells. Comparison of the CML activity after adsorption on various monolayers has revealed that different cytotoxic lymphocytes recognize different alloantigens. This means that individual cytotoxic lymphocytes are not capable of recognizing all alloantigens. It is not known, however, whether individual cytotoxic cells can recognize more than one alloantigen.

V. Genetic Control of CML

The specificity of CML is genetically controlled by the HLA region, which is located on the short arm of chromosome 6. Antigenic disparity, due to differences at the HLA region between responding lymphocytes and stimulating cells, plays an important role in CML, both in the induction of cytotoxic lymphocytes and in the recognition of target cells. Various antigens of the HLA region function differently in these two aspects of CML. Initial studies on the induction of cytotoxic lymphocytes showed a requirement for stimulation by HLA-A and -B antigens as well as by HLA-D antigens. The HLA-D antigens caused strong proliferation in the responding population, and the HLA-A and -B antigens provided the specificity for the reaction. Target cells expressing only the HLA-A and -B antigens could then be recognized by the cytotoxic lymphocytes. More recent studies indicate that stimulation by an HLA-D antigen may not be essential for the induction of cytotoxic lymphocytes. Nevertheless, the CML response may be enhanced if such an HLA-D antigen is presented by the stimulating cell.

Once cytotoxic lymphocytes have been generated they attack target cells in a very specific manner. Early studies indicated that the target determinants recognized by cytotoxic cells are HLA-A or -B antigens. Studies of families with children having recombinant HLA haplotypes revealed that target cells from children who are identical for their HLA-A and -B antigens but different for their HLA-D antigens were recognized in CML, whereas target cells from children identical for the HLA-D antigens but not sharing the HLA-A and -B antigens were not lysed. This indicates either that the antigens recognized by cytotoxic cells are the HLA-A and -B antigens themselves or are controlled by genes closely linked to those genes controlling the HLA-A and -B antigens.

In MLC combinations between unrelated individuals, it was observed that cytotoxic lymphocytes sensitized to several HLA-A and -B antigens could lyse third-party target cells expressing these HLA-A and -B antigens. The cytotoxic lymphocytes, however, showed declining cytotoxic potential for third-party target cells expressing four, three, two, or only one of these sensitizing antigens. In addition, different degrees of CML activity were seen when cytotoxic lymphocytes were sensitized to different HLA-A and -B antigens. For example, several antigens of the HLA-B series seemed to be very potent whereas only certain antigens of the HLA-A series induced strong CML activity. An extensive analysis indicated that if only the HLA-A and -B antigens were important in CML, then they must vary in strength as stimulating and target cell antigens.

In total, these initial studies imply that antigens of the HLA-A and HLA-B series are of qualitative importance in the CML response, but a number of exceptions indicate that other antigens may also be important in CML. In particular, some family studies revealed that target cells from HLA-A and -B identical members were lysed equally by cytotoxic lymphocytes, but third-party target cells obtained from unrelated individuals who express these same HLA-A and -B antigens were damaged to a lesser extent. In unrelated CML combinations, maximum cytotoxicity was observed when cytotoxic lymphocytes were tested against their specific target cells. When third-party target cells from unrelated individuals sharing the same HLA-A and -B antigens were examined, the level of CML lysis was also less.

Additional exceptions to the model that only HLA-A and -B antigens serve as target determinants are apparent from other lines of investigation. First, cytotoxicity has been found in MLC combinations of unrelated individuals identical for their HLA-A and -B antigens. Second, cytotoxic lymphocytes have been found which fail to lyse third-party target cells expressing the same HLA-A and -B antigens to which they have been sensitized. Finally, cytotoxic lymphocytes have been identified that lyse third-party target cells that do not share any HLA-A or -B antigens to which they have been sensitized. These three exceptions indicate an oversimplistic view of the genetic control of CML if only the HLA-A and -B antigens are considered to be of importance. It seems clear that additional determinants must serve as CML sensitizing and target antigens.

New target determinants that are recognized by cytotoxic lymphocytes could either be controlled by genes of the HLA region or determined by genes that segregate independently of this region. Several other antigens known to be controlled by genes of the HLA region would be likely candidates to explain the CML exceptions outlined above. For example, the HLA-C locus controls antigens similar to those of the HLA-A and -B series. Direct evaluation of the role of HLA-C antigens in CML, however, indicates that they are weak both in sensitizing cytotoxic lymphocytes and in serving as target determinants. Antigens controlled by the HLA-D region could also function as target determinants in CML. More recent attempts to detect specific CML responses against these determinants have been successful when bone marrow-derived cells, B-cells, have been used as target cells since these are the predominant lymphocytes expressing HLA-D or HLA-DR antigens. The information on the role of antigens determined by the HLA-C and HLA-D loci is still limited, and thus a complete evaluation can not be made, particularly since many antigens determined by alleles at these two loci have not yet been identified.

Evidence concerning the role of non-HLA determinants also remains unclear. Some studies have reported reactions of cytotoxic lymphocytes to determinants that are not associated with the HLA region, whereas others have found no evidence to indicate that any determinants other than those controlled by the HLA region function in CML.

Interactions between antigens controlled by the HLA region and antigens determined by non-HLA linked genes may provide new determinants that can be recognized by human cytotoxic lymphocytes. An example is the interaction between an HLA-A antigen and the H-Y antigen, controlled by a gene on the human Y chromosome, which can be detected by cytotoxic cells. Again, it will require more extensive analysis of the genetic control of CML to clarify the role of non-HLA gene products, both independently and in conjunction with HLA products.

On the basis of these different observations, the need for means to identify and define new CML target determinants has become apparent. Because of the exquisite specificity that cytotoxic lymphocytes possess for surface determinants on target cells, it has been suggested that they could be used as cellular immunogenetic reagents for defining target cell antigens. The positive cytotoxicity by effector cells of target cells prepared from several unrelated individuals indicates that these third-party target cells share some determinants. Furthermore, cytotoxic lymphocytes generated from different MLC combinations but reacting identically with a panel of target cells are assumed to recognize the same determinant(s) on target cells. Therefore, measurement of the responses of cytotoxic lymphocytes in CML can be used to define target cell determinants.

VI. Cell-Mediated Lympholysis Typing

A method of CML "typing" has been proposed for identifying and defining new target determinants. According to this method, cytotoxic lymphocytes are generated in MLC between allogeneic individuals and tested in CML with panels of third-party target cells. By selecting different combinations of responding and stimulating cells for the MLC, cytotoxic lymphocytes of different specificities are generated. Their specificity is examined by testing them with defined target cell panels. According to the pattern of lysis by one type of cytotoxic lymphocytes, positive and negative groups of target cells are distinguished. Within the positive group, target cells sharing no HLA-A, -B, -C, or -D antigens with the MLC sensitizing cells for the cytotoxic lymphocytes are assumed to express new target determinants.

Table I shows an example of a CML typing experiment. Three different MLC combinations are tested with a panel of 12 cells, including autologous control, specific, and third-party target cells. The first MLC

TABLE I

A Cell-Mediated Lympholysis Typing Experiment[a,b]

MLC combination	Target Cells											
	A*	B*	C*	D*	E*	F*	G*	H*	I*	J*	K*	L*
AA$_x$	0.5	1.8	1.9	1.5	1.4	0.3	0.7	0.6	0.8	0.4	0.2	0.4
AB$_x$	0.4	52.3	45.2	4.1	5.3	5.4	2.2	31.4	3.6	7.9	19.6	35.9
(A3, Bw35, Bw37, Cw4)		A3, Bw35 Bw37, Cw4			Cw4	—		—	—	A3	Cw4 Bw35, Cw4	
AC$_x$	−1.4	56.3	46.1	11.0	11.0	7.6	2.7	37.9	1.9	3.0	21.3	36.8
(B12, Cw5)			B12, Cw5	B12, Cw5	B12	—	—	B12, Cw5	—	—		B12, Cw5

[a] Unpublished observations of D. J. Schendel and R. Wank.

[b] The enclosed values represent those target cells lysed in a similar manner by the cytotoxic lymphocyte combinations AB$_x$ and AC$_x$.

combination, AA_x, does not show any CML activity, demonstrating the requirement for allogeneic sensitization to produce cytotoxic lymphocytes. Both AB_x and AC_x damage some cells of the panel with a high percentage of CML, whereas they cause little or no damage to other target cells. Examination of the pattern of lysis by AB_x alone shows that targets B*, C*, H*, K*, and L* are strongly lysed. Of these five target cells, two cells, C* and H*, do not share any HLA-A, -B, or -C antigens with the B_x stimulating cells. Therefore, they must express a new target determinant recognized by AB_x. The lysis of B*, K*, and L* could be due to recognition of this new antigen as well, but a definite evaluation cannot be made since these three target cells express HLA-A, -B, or -C antigens in common with B_x.

When cells from individual C are used as MLC stimulating cells, a new cytotoxic lymphocyte combination is produced that behaves the same as AB_x. Thus AB_x and AC_x seem to recognize a common determinant in these target cells, a finding that is consistent in a larger analysis of 60 target cells. The same target cells are strongly lysed by AC_x. In this case B* and K* do not share any known HLA antigens with C_x, so their lysis must be due to recognition of a new target determinant. When the information is combined from both cytotoxic lymphocyte combinations it can be concluded that targets B*, C*, H*, and K* share new determinants recognized by both AB_x and AC_x. Therefore, AB_x and AC_x serve as a pair of typing reagents that can identify a new target determinant on these cells that is distinct from defined HLA-A, -B, or -C antigens. Evaluation of the specificity of lysis of target cell L* is still unclear since it shares antigens with both B_x and C_x. Lysis by a third associated cytotoxic lymphocyte combination sensitized to other HLA-A, -B, and -C antigens would be required to analyze this target cell.

Investigations from several laboratories have demonstrated the feasibility of using this approach. Although the concept of CML typing seems to be straightforward, its practical development has been just barely initiated. There are still many problems that must be solved to bring a consequent realization to CML typing.

A. Procurement of Cytotoxic Typing Lymphocytes

Several antigens in the HLA region, including the HLA-A, -B, and -C antigens and possibly new antigens, may be recognized as sensitizing antigens. Therefore cytotoxic lymphocytes of several different specificities will be generated in each allogeneic MLC combination. There is yet no clear means for determining which MLC combinations will be useful in producing cytotoxic lymphocytes recognizing new target determinants. If unrelated individuals, identical for their HLA-A and -B antigens, are used in the MLC, cytotoxic lymphocytes recognizing these antigens will not be generated. The two main difficulties with this approach are that the number of such unrelated combinations available is small and they frequently involve HLA antigens that are in linkage disequilibrium. When genes controlling the HLA-A and -B antigens are in linkage disequilibrium, it is also likely that the genes determining new target determinants will be in linkage disequilibrium with them. Therefore, selecting individuals identical for such HLA-A and -B antigens may result in their being identical for new target determinants. Matching for some of the HLA-A and -B antigens between two unrelated individuals usually is possible. This then limits the sensitizing antigens to be considered and increases the likelihood of identifying cytotoxic lymphocytes specific for new antigens. Since several determinants controlled by each single HLA haplotype may be recognized in CML, restricting MLC sensitization to the differences of one haplotype, using family MLC combinations, may also be useful.

B. Standardized Target Cell Panels

Large numbers of target cells must be tested in CML to characterize the specificity of cytotoxic lymphocytes. The use of cryopreserved lymphocytes as target cells is very useful, allowing procurement and storage of cells from large numbers of individuals. The cells of this target panel should be well characterized for their HLA-A, -B, and -C antigens, and information on their HLA-D and -DRw specificities is also helpful for analyzing the specificity of cytotoxic lymphocytes. Cryopreservation of cells from all members of HLA typed families is valuable for segregation studies.

C. Definition of Positive and Negative Responses

The level of cytotoxicity between cytotoxic lymphocytes and specific target cells varies from experiment to experiment, making it difficult to compare data directly. Several CML experiments must be done to test a panel of target cells obtained from 50–100 unrelated individuals, when only 10–20 different target cells can be analyzed in one experiment. It has, therefore, been suggested that calculation of CML data according to a relative cytotoxic response may be useful. This method defines the specific percentage of CML (i.e., $AB_x + B^{51}Cr$) as a reference value of 100% and expresses the lysis of a third-party target cell (i.e., $Y^{51}Cr$) as a percentage of this response. This calculation is designated as the relative cytotoxic response (RCR) and is determined as follows:

$$\% \text{ Relative Cytotoxic Response} = \frac{\% \text{ CML of } AB_x + Y^{51}Cr}{\% \text{ CML of } AB_x + B^{51}Cr} \times 100.$$

According to the results of a recent study, an RCR of 10% could be used to distinguish negative and positive responses. Nevertheless, a major problem remains in understanding the specificity of the CML response when positive values vary from 10 to 100% RCR.

D. Analysis of the Specificity of Cytotoxic Lymphocytes

Once cytotoxic lymphocytes have been tested with the target cell panel, certain information regarding their specificity can be analyzed. It should be demonstrated that no HLA-A, -B, or -C antigens are expressed by all the target cells that are significantly lysed by the cytotoxic lymphocytes. This is most easily done by a computer program, comparing each of the antigens of the HLA-A, -B, and -C series with the group of positive target cells. When cytotoxic lymphocytes of only one type are tested with the panel, none of the target cells sharing an HLA-A, -B, or -C antigen with the MLC sensitizing cells can be clearly assigned the new determinant. Lysis of these target cells may be due either to the recognition of the new determinant or of a shared HLA-A, -B, or -C antigen. If two or more different cytotoxic lymphocyte combinations can be found giving very similar results on the panel, they most likely recognize similar target determinants. When these different combinations have been generated in MLC using cells from individuals expressing different HLA-A, -B, and -C antigens, then most target cells can be evaluated. Recognition by two associated cytotoxic lymphocytes means the target cells most likely express the new target determinant.

To examine the role of HLA-D or -DRw antigens as target determinants, one can compare the expression of these antigens on the positive target cells of the panel. Many target cells, however, may have only one, or perhaps neither, of the HLA-D specificities identified. Direct evaluation of the role of HLA-D and -DRw antigens can be made by comparing subpopulations of lymphocytes as target cells. Since the HLA-D and -DRw antigens are primarily expressed on bone marrow-derived (B) lymphocytes, cytotoxic lymphocytes specific for these determinants would be expected to lyse subpopulations of B lymphocytes but not of thymus-derived (T) lymphocytes.

It is also important to study segregation patterns in families to determine whether the cytotoxic lymphocytes recognize determinants controlled by the HLA region. If the MLC sensitizing cells for cytotoxic lymphocytes express HLA-A, -B, or -C antigens present in a family, then CML responses to these antigens may interfere with the analysis of the new determinants. Occasionally it may be possible to find cytotoxic lymphocytes that recognize a new determinant in a family but have not been sensitized to shared HLA-A, -B, or -C antigens. If several cytotoxic lymphocytes, prepared from different MLC combinations but showing associations in their specificity, are available, they may allow demonstration of segregation with or without the HLA region. Having demonstrated that one particular cytotoxic lymphocyte combination identifies a new target determinant that is not an HLA-A, -B, -C, -D, or -DRw determinant, there remains a difficulty in using it as a typing reagent, since it may still recognize more than one new target determinant. Again, it is important to identify associated cytotoxic lymphocyte combinations that are sensitized to different HLA-A, -B, and -C antigens and to seem to recognize one common new determinant. In the future, it may be possible to clone individual cytotoxic lymphocytes in order to obtain cells specific for one determinant.

E. Selection of Cells Identical for New Target Specificities

If enough cytotoxic lymphocytes can be identified that recognize new and different target determinants, it may be possible to use them to identify cells in the target panel that are identical for new target antigens. If normal peripheral blood lymphocytes from the donors of these target cells are then mutually sensitized against each other in MLC and tested in CML, it will be possible to evaluate the role of these antigens in the *in vitro* CML response. By this means it may be possible to assess the relationships between different cell surface antigens in their strength for sensitizing cytotoxic cells and for serving as target antigens.

VII. Preliminary Information from CML Typing Experiments

To date, over 30 combinations of different cytotoxic lymphocytes have been identified that seem to recognize new target determinants. Some of these individual cytotoxic combinations have been extensively analyzed. A number of them show associations to HLA-A, -B, or -C antigens, revealing that the target cells that are recognized by the cytotoxic lymphocytes frequently, although not always, express particular HLA-A or -B antigens. Such associations indicate that the new target determinants are in some way connected with the HLA region. This could be due to recognition by the cytotoxic lymphocytes of a determinant on the same molecule as the HLA-A or -B antigens, or the new target determinant and the HLA-A or -B antigen may be associated on the membrane. Such an association could also be seen if the genes controlling the new determinant and the HLA-A or -B antigens are in linkage disequilibrium in the population and would therefore frequently occur together in unrelated individuals. If the third explanation is correct, then the finding that some cytotoxic lymphocytes show associations to HLA-A antigens whereas others show associations to HLA-B antigens indicates that at least two genes may govern these new target determinants.

Segregation studies indicate that some new target determinants follow the HLA haplotype inheritance patterns in families. A recent study has revealed that the new determinant recognized by two associated cytotoxic lymphocyte combinations was determined by complementation effects by two HLA haplotypes within a family. Thus inheritance of a single HLA haplotype did not lead to expression of the new target determinant, but the inheritance of two particular HLA haplotypes did. Such patterns reveal that gene interactions or interactions of molecules at the cell surface may influence recognition in CML. Therefore in analyzing the specificity of cytotoxic lymphocytes, it must be kept in mind that not only can one HLA haplotype determine several target cell antigens, but also interactions between two different HLA haplotypes may influence their specificity.

An exchange among laboratories of approximately 30 cytotoxic lymphocyte "typing" combinations enabled testing of a panel of 100 third-party unrelated target cells, obtained from a Danish population. This analysis yielded very surprising and encouraging information since the cytotoxic lymphocytes could be divided into three different groups, which showed similar patterns of lysis of the target cell panel. Therefore, by testing only this small number of different typing combinations, it was possible to find associated groups of cytotoxic lymphocytes that seemed to recognize similar determinants. In the future, it may be reasonable to assume that additional clusters of cytotoxic typing cells will be identified and that these reagents can be utilized as a genetic tool for defining histocompatibility antigens.

VIII. Future Prospects

Matching for HLA-A, -B, and -C antigens in donor–recipient pairs for transplantation has been very successful in families, but of only limited value in unrelated individuals. Therefore, there is considerable interest in developing rapid and sensitive tests that can define other alloantigens important in the process of graft rejection. For example, antigens of the HLA-D region that stimulate lymphocyte proliferation may be significant in causing graft rejection. Development of serological and cellular techniques, such as B cell typing and primed lymphocyte typing, will allow rapid identification of these antigens so that they particularly may be used in transplant situations using cadaver organs.

Since cytotoxic lymphocytes are found in the circulation of allotransplant recipients during graft rejection crises, it is assumed that these cells play a role in the rejection process. In some cases, even though the donor and recipient have been matched for their HLA-A, -B, -C, and -D antigens, circulating cytotoxic cells have been observed. Therefore, recognition of other allogeneic determinants must activate this destructive activity of the immune system. This observation emphasizes the importance of studying the CML response in donor–recipient pairs. When living related individuals are used as organ transplant donors, it is possible to study cytotoxic responses in the indirect CML assay with the donor and recipient. In the case of cadaveric organ transplantation, however, the 6-day time period of the assay prohibits this analysis. CML typing provides a rapid means for identifying and defining new target determinants. Since cytotoxic typing cell combinations can be cryopreserved, it is feasible to perform CML typing in only a few hours, making this analysis applicable to the cadaveric organ transplant situation as well.

Our increased understanding of the complexity of the genetic control of cell-mediated cytotoxicity requires a reevaluation of the role of various gene products controlled by the HLA region as targets for CML. It may be demonstrated that only some antigens are recognized predominantly by cytotoxic lymphocytes, and perhaps these may be the new determinants identified by CML typing. In the future, therefore, selection of transplant pairs identical for these determinants may be possible. If matching for such new antigens does not solve the problems of graft rejection completely, it is hoped that it may add another increment to the number of successful transplants.

In order to develop the means to type for new determinants and select matched individuals, certain basic information must be obtained. The nature of the genetic system controlling these antigens must be understood, including identification of the number of genes involved and their degree of polymorphism. The location of these genes must be studied to find out whether they are located in the HLA region, on chromosome 6, or, perhaps, even on different chromosomes. The relationship of these new target determinants to other antigens controlled by the HLA region must be investigated to understand their association, not only at the genetic level, but also at the level of expression on the cell surface. Such information will allow a better understanding of the genetic complexity of the HLA region and its role in the control of the allograft response. Only the answers to some of these basic questions will determine the feasibility of finding individuals who are identical, or at least similar, for cytotoxic target determinants.

Although the current emphasis in CML typing is directed toward the identification of alloantigens that may lead to graft rejection, it is possible at some later date that cytotoxic lymphocytes specific for tumor antigens might also be identified. Such cells could then be used to define tumor-specific antigens and perhaps even be used as immunotherapeutic agents to mediate specific damage to tumor cells.

Suggested Reading List[2]

Technical References

Kristensen, T., Grunnet, N., Jorgensen, F., Lamm, L., and Kissmeyer-Nielsen, F. (1976). Cell mediated lympholysis in man. An attempt to type with cytotoxic lymphocytes. *Tissue Antigens* **8,** 299–316.

Lightbody, J., Bernoco, D., Miggiano, V. C., and Ceppellini, R. (1971). Cell mediated lympholysis in man after sensitization of effector lymphocytes through mixed leukocyte cultures. *G. Batteriol. Virol. Immunol. Ann. Osp. Maria Vittoria Torino* **64,** 243–254.

Schendel, D. J., Wank, R., and Dupont, B. (1979). Standardization of the human *in vitro* cell-mediated lympholysis technique. *Tissue Antigens* **13,** 112–120.

Review Articles

Albert, E., and Götze, D. (1977). The major histocompatibility system in man. *In* "The Major Histocompatibility System in Man and Animals" (D. Götze, ed.), pp. 7–77. Springer-Verlag, Berlin.

Bach, F. H., and van Rood, J. J. (1976). The major histocompatibility complex—genetics and biology. *N. Engl. J. Med.* **295,** 872–878.

Dupont, B., Hansen, J. A., and Yunis, E. J. (1976). Human mixed-lymphocyte culture reaction: Genetics, specificity, and biological implications. *Adv. Immunol.* **23,** 107–202.

Eijsvoogel, V. P., Schellekens, P. T. A., Du Bois, M. J. G. J., and Zeijlemaker, W. P. (1976). Human cytotoxic lymphocytes after alloimmunization *in vitro*. *Transplant. Rev.* **29,** 125–145.

Kristensen, T. (1978). Studies on the specificity of CML. Report from CML-Workshop. *Tissue Antigens* **11,** 330–349.

---

[2] In agreement with the general policy of this volume, only technical references and review articles are cited.

HLA and Graft Survival[1]

J. J. VAN ROOD and G. G. PERSIJN

Department of Immunohematology University Medical Center, Leiden,
The Netherlands, and Eurotransplant Foundation, Leiden, The Netherlands

I. Introduction	161
II. Methodology	164
III. Results	166
IV. Discussion	170
References	171

I. Introduction

Systematic studies on the influence of HLA matching on graft survival have been carried out for more than 15 years, but it is only quite recently that these studies produced significant, although still only partial, information. This does not imply that the role of HLA in determining graft survival was not established long ago, for this was done already in 1964, but insight as to the role of the different HLA determinants in graft survival is of very recent date.

That the HLA region and its equivalent in other species carried information of overriding importance in graft survival was established

---

[1] This work was supported in part by the Dutch Foundation for Medical Research (FUNGO), which is subsidized by the Dutch Organization for the Advancement of Pure Research (ZWO); the Dutch Organization for Health Research (TNO); and the J. A. Cohen Institute for Radiopathology and Radiation Protection (IRS) and the Dutch Kidney Foundation.

first with the help of experimental skin grafts and later for kidney and other grafts. The protocol was simple: graft survival for grafts exchanged between HLA-identical donor–recipient sibling pairs was compared with graft survival of HLA-nonidentical sibling pairs. The information was clear-cut and reproducible in many different centers and was highly significant in indicating the improved survival with HLA identity (Tables I and II and Fig. 1). This established beyond all rea-

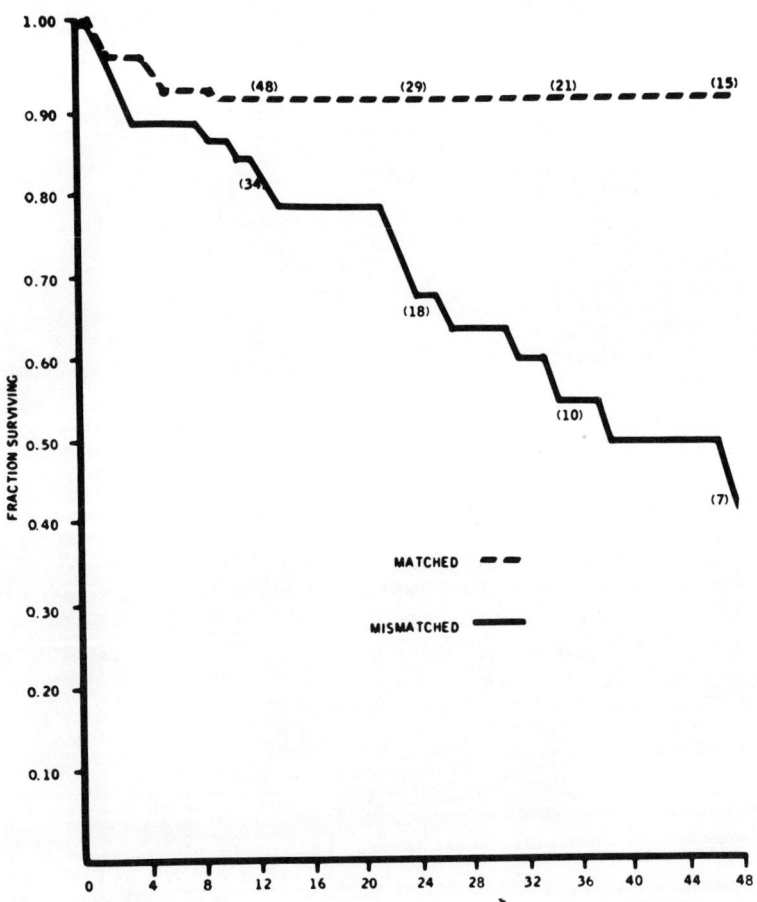

Fig. 1. Kidneys from HLA-identical sibling donors (- - -) survive significantly longer than those from HLA-incompatible ones (———). Abscissa, days. (From Singal *et al.*, 1969.)

TABLE I
SKIN GRAFT REJECTION TIMES IN SIBLINGS

	Days (mean ± SE)	N
HLA identical	24.9 ± 1.1	43
One haplotype different	14.4 ± 0.34	115
Two haplotypes different	11.6 ± 0.54	18

a Adapted from Amos *et al.* (1969).

sonable doubt that the HLA system was a major factor in determining graft survival in ABO-compatible donor–recipient combinations.

This last restriction has to be made because the ABO system is an important transplantation antigen system on its own account for kidney and skin grafts, but curiously enough not in bone marrow transplantation. We will not discuss this topic further here.

That this information was incomplete became clear when it was applied to matching for cadaveric renal transplantation between unrelated donor–recipient pairs. Results even between HLA-A and -B-identical unrelated donor–recipient pairs was significantly poorer than between HLA-identical sibling pairs. This led to statements of some workers that matching for HLA in unrelated donor–recipient pairs is of only borderline importance, a statement that is in direct contradiction with the general accepted role of HLA in sibling combinations. In retro-

TABLE II
EFFICACY OF HLA MATCHING IN BONE MARROW GRAFTING

	Bone marrow donors	
	HLA-identical	HLA-nonidentical
Alive	6	2
Dead	5	14

a Based on data collected and published by Buckley (1971).

b In a worldwide survey it could be shown that bone marrow grafts from HLA-identical sibling donors are to be preferred when the immune potential in immune-deficient children must be restored. Only cases in which a bone marrow graft was certain or likely have been included.

spect, this contradiction can be understood by the realization that even now in unrelated combinations only partial matching for HLA is possible (i.e., we can recognize only certain markers of HLA), in contrast to the situation in siblings, where matching for HLA implies identity not only for the markers one can recognize, but also for those for which detection is not yet possible. Partial identity implies partial incompatibility, and this incompatibility might provide "help" for non-HLA systems, which without this help might be only weakly immunogenic.

The disappointing results of HLA matching in cadaveric renal transplantation led to many retro- and prospective studies.

II. Methodology

The role of HLA on graft survival has been studied with the help of three basic approaches: (a) experimental grafts in man (skin) and animals; (b) retrospective studies of clinical kidney and to a lesser extent bone marrow transplants; (c) studies on *in vitro* cell interactions. None of these studies would have been possible without the work on HLA in man and related systems in other species.

Experimental skin grafts in man became possible after Rapaport and Converse developed a standardized procedure with objective criteria to establish the occurrence of graft rejection (Converse and Rapaport, 1956). With only minor adaptations this method has been used by all workers in the field. The method consists of the transplantation of a circular full-thickness skin graft to a recipient on whom a site has been prepared by removing not full-thickness skin, but only split skin. Rejection, as evidenced by hemorrhages and edema, can be objectively ascertained with the help of a stereomicroscope. Skin graft survival is measured in days and is approximately 10 days for grafts transplanted between unrelated donor–recipient pairs selected at random; this is an obvious advantage if one wants to evaluate the effectiveness of matching procedures. Survival is influenced by immunization of the recipient and the presence of grafts from multiple donors instead of a single donor. Skin grafts, for obvious reasons, are the only experimental grafts that can be used in man, but in other species survival of other grafts could be studied as well. Here the information from species such as nonhuman primates and dogs have been particularly useful (Fig. 2).

Retrospective studies especially of renal transplants in man have so far provided the most critical information. It is obvious that this kind

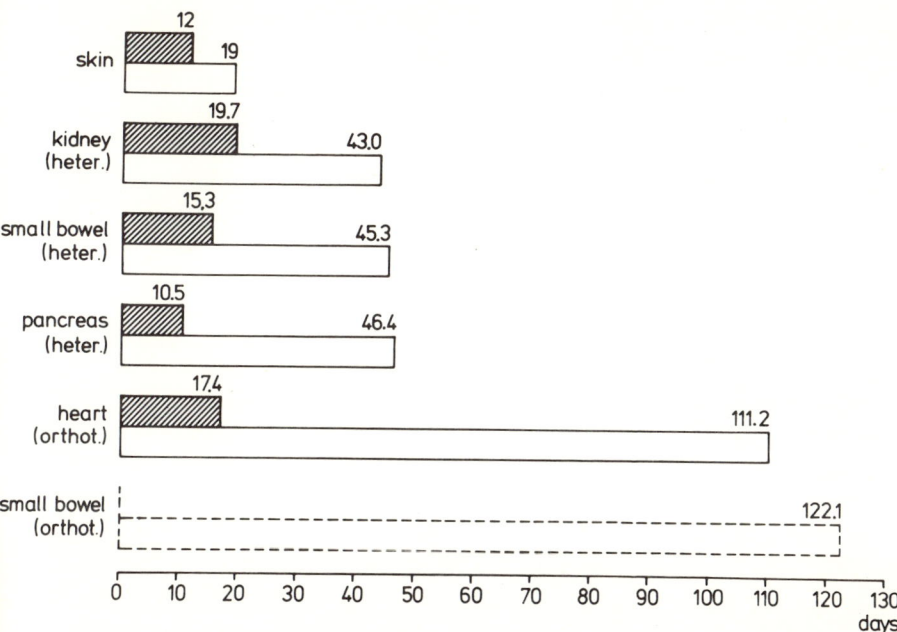

Fig. 2. Summary of experimental organ grafts in beagle dogs. Mean survival times of different allografts in identical and nonidentical lettermates (without immunosuppressive therapy). ▨, 1 or 2 DL-A haplotype differences; ☐, no haplotype differences; heter. heterotropic; orthot., orthotopic. Note the difference in rejection time for the different organs. (From Vriesendorp *et al.*, 1973.)

of analysis carries many risks. A double-blind trial on the importance of HLA matching has not been performed in the true sense of the word. Most centers tried to get the best possible match for their patients, whereas a few did not bother at all. Many analyses concerned—in view of the large numbers of variables influencing graft survival—relatively small numbers of patients, and many were subjected to a procedure of analysis that was at least in part incorrect. As Peto *et al.* (1977) pointed out, when two sets of data (e.g., graft survival in two different groups of patients) are followed, significant differences in, for instance, graft survival can occur in the third month after transplantation. It is quite correct to denote this as significant, if it is indeed significant. It should be realized, however, that after 3 months there are two possibilities. One is that the difference in graft survival of the two groups is the same after, e.g., 6 months as after, e.g., 3 months. If the numbers are large enough, the difference of the survival rate will remain significant. The rejection rate of the two groups is in fact the same. On the other hand, if graft rejection after 3 months becomes larger in one group than in the other, either the significance can be lost (i.e., if the "good" starts to fail) or it can become greater. In summary the significance of the rate of change between two or more actuarial curves should be differentiated from the significance of the difference of the proportion surviving at any point on the curve.

Finally, the *in vitro* test of cellular interaction had an enormous impact on our understanding of the role of the HLA system in graft rejection. The introduction of the mixed lymphocyte culture (MLC) test by Bach and Bain visualized what could happen if lymphocytes of two individuals met during, for instance, a reaction to an organ transplant. The introduction of what is now called the cell-mediated lympholysis (CML) test by Haÿry and Defendi and Svedmyr and Hodes in mouse and by Solliday and Rich in man and its adaptation by Lightbody, Miggiano, and Ceppellini for easy use in man provided a test that until now is considered to be the best *in vitro* equivalent of the homograft reaction (see chapter on CML testing by Schendel in this volume).

III. Results

That matching for the HLA-A and -B antigens (insufficient information is available for HLA-C), not only between sibling donor–recipient pairs, but also between unrelated individuals can improve graft survival has been established beyond any reasonable doubt. This was first established in individuals who had been immunized against certain HLA antigens. Skin and kidney grafts carrying these incompatible antigens were rejected much earlier as compared to grafts from donors who lacked these antigens. From these observations originated the rule that no kidney should be transplanted if it had not first been established that the serum of the prospective recipient did not contain antibodies that could react with the donor's lymphocytes. But also in nonimmunized individuals, HLA matching can improve graft survival, as shown in Table III, which contains the results of skin graft data collected by our group as analyzed by Jonker. Although the difference is not impressive, it is consistent and quite significant. That these experimental data were also relevant for clinical renal transplantation is illustrated in Fig. 3. It depicts kidney graft survival at 5 years in Eurotransplant in more than 3000 donor–recipient combinations. In the

TABLE III
INFLUENCE OF MATCHING FOR HLA-A, -B, AND MIXED LEUKOCYTE CULTURE (MLC) ON SKIN GRAFT SURVIVAL

Donor–recipient combination			Mean ± SD	N
HLA-A, −B	=	MLC+	10.40 ± 1.19	20
HLA-A, −B	=	MLC+	11.80 ± 0.89	20
HLA-A, −B	=	MLC−	15.57 ± 1.53	3
HLA-A, −B	=	MLC−	17.25 ± 2.50	4

[a] Adapted from Jonker et al. (1978).

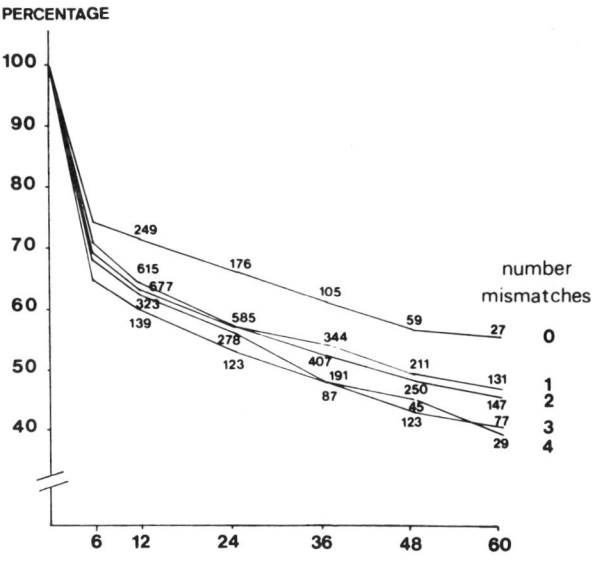

Fig. 3. Kidney graft survival in 3002 consecutive transplants performed in collaboration with the Eurotransplant organ exchange organization. Note that after 6 months there is an 8% difference and after 60 months a 15% difference between the best and poorest matched grafts. (From Persijn et al., 1979.)

full-house identical group this was 60% versus 40% in those mismatched for 4 HLA-A and -B antigens. The difference in graft survival already became significant after 6 months. Whether the kidneys were mismatched for 1 or 2 antigens did not appear to make too much difference. We will want to return to this point later. Similar findings have been reported by most European centers and, although often less striking, by several centers in the United States.

Although there is thus no doubt that matching for HLA-A and -B can improve survival of grafts exchanged between unrelated donor–recipient pairs, it is equally clear that even when donor and recipient were HLA-A and -B identical graft survival was significantly poorer than that obtained between HLA-identical sibling pairs.

Many different explanations were considered (influence of HLA-C, incomplete typing and thus matching for HLA-A and -B, etc.), but the assumption that structures other than HLA-A, -B, and -C, i.e., the MLC stimulating determinants, influenced graft survival quite significantly was favored by most workers from the beginning. Preliminary evidence to support this was first presented for kidney grafts in related donor–recipient combinations by Hamburger, Jeannet, and Russell. Experimental skin graft studies provided further information (Table III). It appeared that MLC-negative but HLA-A- and -B incompatible skin grafts survived longer than did MLC-positive but HLA-A- and -B-identical grafts, and MLC-negative HLA-A- and -B-identical grafts survived best. These data strongly suggest that selecting MLC-negative donor–recipient combinations might be a better way to improve graft survival than matching for HLA-A and -B alone, if matching for both cannot be realized. Cochrum presented retrospective data of cadaveric renal transplantation that were in agreement with the skin graft findings.

These findings put an obvious challenge before those involved in clinical organ transplantation: to find ways and means to select donor–recipient combinations with a low or negative MLC. This is sometimes feasible when living donors are available, but becomes an enormous logistic problem when only cadaveric donors are available. The MLC test itself takes too long; other selection procedures have been proposed but are not operational (see discussion of primed LD typing by Bach and Sondel in this volume). These considerations provided a strong stimulus to develop what is now called HLA-DR typing. As outlined in the review on the serology of HLA-DR by van Rood and van Leeuwen in this volume, this method is now available, and it is possible to select unrelated individuals who are HLA-DR identical. Because of the limited polymorphism of DR, this is relatively easy. Incidently, about 50% of the donor–recipient combinations in Eurotransplant (i.e., with selection for, at least partial, HLA-A and -B identity) share one HLA-DR determinant.

To investigate the importance of HLA-DR matching in kidney transplantation, our group performed a retrospective study which showed that kidney graft survival was improved when donor and recipient share 1 or 2 HLA-DR antigens. Similar observations have been made by Morris, Thoeby, Festenstein, and Jeannet. All of these studies were criticized because typing for the HLA-DR determinants was not done prospectively. To meet this criticism, patients on the Eurotransplant waiting list were typed prospectively for HLA-DR. Kidney donors were HLA-DR typed before or at time of transplantation.

Figure 4 shows that 90% graft survival is obtained if kidney donor and recipient are not HLA-DR mismatched. In the retrospectively typed patients there is a clearcut difference in kidney graft survival between the group with one HLA-DR mismatch and those with two HLA-DR mismatches namely 80% versus 60% after 6 months. This

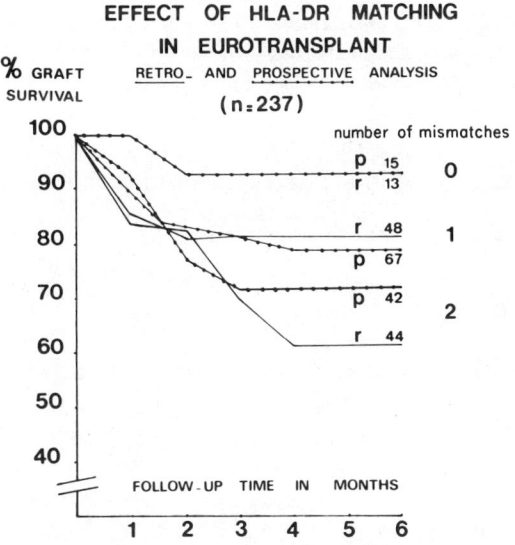

Fig. 4. The effect of HLA-DR matching in Eurotransplant (numbers are the patients at risk; p = prospectively typed; r = retrospectively typed). (From Persijn *et al.*, 1979.)

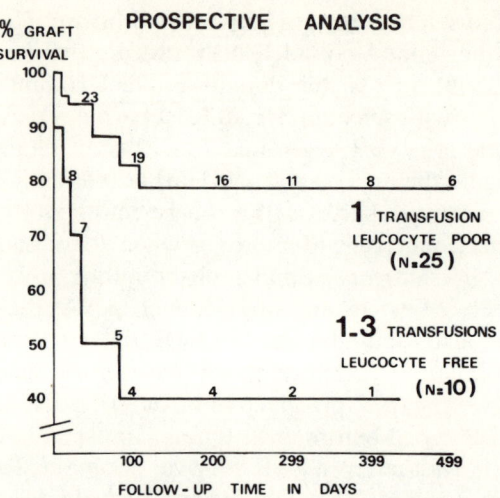

Fig. 5. Kidney graft survival in prospectively transfused patients (numbers are the patients at risk). (From Persijn *et al.*, 1979.)

difference is less outspoken in the prospectively typed group namely 77% versus 70%.

All patients recieved pretransplant blood transfusions. Many investigators have shown that pretransplant blood transfusions improve kidney graft survival. However, the mechanism by which blood transfusion improve kidney graft survival is not clearly understood. Persijn *et al.* (1979) have shown that even one leucocyte-poor blood transfusion, sometimes given a long time before transplantation, is sufficient to improve kidney graft survival (Fig. 5).

IV. Discussion

The data reviewed in this chapter clearly indicate that many different factors influence kidney graft survival: ABO-compatibility, HLA-A, -B., and -DR matching and pretransplant blood transfusion(s).

Obviously the combination of pretransplant blood transfusion(s), immunosupppression and matching for the HLA-A, -B and -DR antigens facilitates the induction of specific nonresponsiveness vis-a-vis the kidney graft. It is generally accepted that differences for HLA-DR can trigget the immune response by activating helper cells. Thereafter, humoral and cellular immune activity against the graft will occur. The fact that matching for the HLA-DR determinants improves kidney graft survival significantly is in accordance with this. One would expect that complete matching for HLA-A and -B without matching for HLA-DR would also improve kidney graft survival in a significant manner. This is generally not the case. Although improvement of graft survival is observed, it is generally not more than the 15% between best matched and poorly matched grafts (Fig. 3). One possible explanation might be that kidney graft is not primarily rejected via humoral or cellular immune activity against the HLA-A and -B antigens themselves, but against other antigenic systems. The endothelial-monocyte antigens recently described by Paul *et al.* could be relevant here.

For an understanding of the role of blood transfusions in renal transplantation, one must appreciate the preliminary findings in monkey and man indicating that pretransplant blood transfusions in recipients who receive an HLA-DR identical kidney have almost no additive beneficial effect on kidney graft survival. The observations by Balner, Morris, and Van Rood and Persijn suggest that the beneficial effect of blood transfusions may work through blockage of the detrimental effects of differences for the HLA-D antigens between donor and recipients. Whether this blocking is due to enhancement or an other mechanism remains to be assessed. The fact that only one blood transfusion produces a beneficial effect on graft survival indicates that the blocking antibodies, if any, must have a very broad specificity.

The enthusiasm induced by the easily attainable and, apparently, effective DR matching should not let us forget that many factors influencing graft survival are sufficiently understood or identified. For instance, incompatibility for the red cell Lewis system can, according to some people, interfere with graft survival. Also, the influence of the HLA-A, -B, and -DR antigens and the above-mentioned endothelial-monocyte antigens demand further analysis. Undoubtedly, the study of histocompatibility antigens and organ transplantation and its outcome will remain a fascinating field for many years to come.

References

Amos, D. B., Seigler, H. F., Southworth, J. G., and Ward, F. E. (1969). *Transplant. Proc.* **I,** 1 (Pt. II), 342.
Bach, F. H., and van Rood, J. J. (1976). *N. Engl. J. Med.* **295,** 806, 872, 927.

Buckley, R. H. (1971). *In* "Progress in Immunology" (D. B. Amos, ed.), Academic Press, New York, p. 1061.
Ceppellini, R., Mattiuz, P. L., Scudeller, G., and Visetti, M. (1969). *Transplant. Proc.* **I,** 1 (Pt. II), 385.
Converse, J. H., and Rapaport, F. T. (1956). *Ann. Surg.* **143,** 306.
Jonker, M., Hoogeboom, J., van Leeuwen, A., Koch, C. T., Blussé van Oud Alblas, A., Persijn, G. G., Fredriks, E., and van Rood, J. J. (1979). *Transplant. Proc.* **XI,** 607.
Merrell, M., and Shulman, L. E. (1955). *J. Chron. Dis.* **1,** 12.
Persijn, G. G., van Leeuwen, A., Nagtegaal, A., Hoogeboom, J., and van Rood, J. J. (1978). *Lancet* **1,** 1278.
Persijn, G. G., Cohen, B., Lansberge, Q., and van Rood, J. J. (1979). *Transplantation* **20,** 5,396.
Peto, R., Pike, M. C., Armitage, P., Breslow, N. E., Cox, D. R., Howard, S. V., Mantel, N., McPherson, K., Peto, J., and Smith, P. G. (1977). *Br. J. Cancer* **35,** 1.
Singal, D. P., Mickey, M. R., and Terasaki, P. I. (1969). *Transplantation* **7,** 4, 246.
van Es, A. A., and Balner, H. (1979). *Transplantation* **20,** 2, 135.
van Rood, J. J., Blussé van Oud Alblas, A., Keuning, J. J., Frederiks, E., Termijtelen, A., van Hooff, J. P., Peña, A. S., and van Leeuwen, A. (1975). *Transplant. Proc.* **VII,** 25.
van Rood, J. J., Persijn, G. G., van Leeuwen, A., Goulmy, E., and Gabb, B. W. (1979). *Transplant. Proc.* **XI,** 736.
Vriesendorp, H. M., D'Amaro, J., van der Does, J. A., Westbroek, D. L., and Epstein, R. B. (1973). *Transplant. Proc.* **V,** 1, 311.
Williams, U. A., Ting. A., Cullen, P. R, and Morris. P. J. (1979). *Transplant. Proc.* **XI,** 175.

HLA and Disease

A. SVEJGAARD and L. P. RYDER

*HLA and Disease Registry, Tissue-Typing Laboratory,
State University Hospital of Copenhagen (Rigshospitalet), Copenhagen, Denmark*

I. Introduction	173
II. Methods	174
III. Relationships between HLA and Diseases	175
IV. Disease Heterogeneity	176
V. Inheritance of Disease Susceptibility and Resistance	177
VI. Mechanisms that Can Explain the Associations	179
VII. Diagnostic and Prognostic Value	180
Key References	181

I. Introduction

The HLA system in man was originally discovered as a leukocyte blood group system, and the next important discovery was the identification of HLA as the human major histocompatibility complex (MHC), which controls the strongest transplantation antigens of the species. However, probably the most far reaching discovery in this area of research was the surprising demonstration in the early 1970s that the HLA system is deeply involved in the development of a variety of diseases with largely unknown etiology and pattern of inheritance. The detection of these relationships is a major breakthrough in human genetics because they make it possible to study the inheritance of disease susceptibility and resistance in much more detail than was previously possible. In addition, they have considerable prospects in the unraveling of the etiologies and pathogeneses of the disorders in question, and they have already been useful in distinguishing between various subgroups of diseases. In a few cases, the relationships are even so strong that HLA typing has become a diagnostic aid. The purpose of this review is to summarize some of the most important connections between HLA and disease and to outline how this knowledge may be applied in terms of nosology, genetics, pathogenesis, and diagnosis.

II. Methods

Relationships between HLA and diseases may be established by both population and family studies. In population studies it is investigated whether one or more HLA characters occur with different frequencies in a group of unrelated patients as compared to the corresponding frequencies in healthy, unrelated individuals of the same ethnic group. If this is the case, there is association between the HLA factors in question and the disease. Table I illustrates the analysis of the 2 × 2 table obtained when comparing the frequency of the HLA-Dw2 antigen in patients with multiple sclerosis. The strength of the association is estimated by the so-called "relative risk," which indicates how many times more frequently the diseases occurs in HLA-Dw2-positive individuals as compared to HLA-Dw2 negative ones. In this case, HLA-Dw2-positives have 4.3 times as high a risk as Dw2-negatives. The statistical significance is evaluated by the well known chi square test or by Fisher's exact method, both of which yield highly significant p values, as shown in Table I. Usually, more than 20 different HLA antigens are compared between patients and controls, and accordingly there is a considerable possibility that the frequency for one of these

TABLE I
ASSOCIATION BETWEEN HLA-Dw2 AND MULTIPLE SCLEROSIS[a]

Individuals	Dw2-positive	Dw2-negative	Total
Multiple sclerosis	58 (60%)	39	97
Controls	89 (26%)	256	345

[a] Relative risk: $(58 \times 256)/(39 \times 89) = 4.3$.
Statistical significance: $\chi^2 = 37.9$ with 1 df $\sim p < 10^{-8}$; Fisher's exact $p = 10^{-9}$.

may deviate by chance alone. Hence, the usual significance limits cannot be used in these studies, but more conservative ones (p values well below 0.1%) must be applied.

Family studies are usually more complicated than population studies both from a practical point of view, because the relatives are often scattered, and in terms of analysis. The major principle is to investigate whether affected relatives share HLA haplotypes more often than they would according to the classical genetic rules. These investigations are linkage studies of a sort, but when they concern conditions characterized by incomplete penetrance and varying age at onset, the analysis become even more difficult, and it would lead too far to discuss these methods here.

III. Relationships between HLA and Diseases

A large number of the most diverse diseases have already been studied in terms of HLA. Many of these studies have yielded negative or inconclusive results, but a surprising number of diseases have been found to show definite relationships to the HLA system. In Table II we have listed the most representative of these disorders. It can be seen that they span from rheumatology over neurology, dermatology, and immunopathology to endocrinology. However, it is a striking fact that no malignancies have shown strong relationships to HLA. The majority of the relationships have been found in population studies, and in these cases we have indicated the associated HLA antigen(s), the frequency of this antigen in healthy Caucasians (a Danish population has been used as reference) and in Caucasian patients, and the relative risk. However, two disorders (both clear-cut recessive traits) were first found to be HLA related in family studies: complement factor 2 (C2) deficiency and congenital adrenal hyperplasia due to 21-hydroxylase deficiency. The first of these also shows a very strong association to HLA; in fact, almost all patients with C2 deficiency, who are homozygous for the $C2^0$ deficiency gene, are also homozygous for the *HLA-Dw2* gene, which shows that the *C2* gene by definition is part of the HLA system. In analogy, the gene for 21-hydroxylase deficiency has also been mapped within the HLA complex, and most recently, an association between this disorder and HLA-Bw47 has been found.

TABLE II
RELATIONSHIPS BETWEEN HLA AND DISEASE

Disease	Associated HLA antigen	Frequency (%) of antigen		Relative risk
		Controls	Patients	
Ankylosing spondylitis	B27	8.6	89	90.1
Reiter's syndrome	B27	8.6	77	35.9
Acute anterior uveitis	B27	8.6	47	9.4
Rheumatoid arthirits	Dw4	19.4	48	3.9
Multiple sclerosis	Dw2	25.8	60	4.3
Myasthenia gravis	B8	23.7	56	4.1
Celiac disease	Dw3	26.3	96	73.0
Dermatitis herpetiformis	Dw3	26.3	83	13.5
Chronic autoimmune hepatitis	Dw3	26.3	71	6.8
Sicca syndrome	Dw3	26.3	87	19.0
Idiopathic Addison's disease	Dw3	26.3	76	8.8
Graves' disease	Dw3	26.3	61	4.4
Insulin-dependent diabetes	Dw2	25.8	0	0.0
	Dw3	26.3	48	2.5
	Dw4	19.4	49	3.9
Subacute thyroiditis	Bw35	13.1	72	16.8
Psoriasis vulgaris	Cw6	33.1	88	14.9
Idiopathic hemachromatosis	A3	26.9	73	7.4
	B14	4.5	19	5.0
C2 deficiency	Strongly associated with Dw2, in particular the *A25*, *B18*, *Dw2* haplotype			
Congential adrenal hyperplasia (21-hydroxylase deficiency)	Closely linked to HLA and associated with HLA-Bw47			

IV. Disease Heterogeneity

One important aspect of the relationships listed in Table II is that they have permitted a more precise distinction between various subgroups of disease entities. For example, it has long been a matter of debate whether juvenile-onset and maturity-onset diabetes were one and the same or two different diseases. Now, the fact that only the juvenile form shows association with HLA, whereas the late-onset form does not, confirms the latter notion. Moreover, it seems as though insulin dependency is a better criterion when distinguishing between the two forms than is the age at onset. In analogy, the earlier clinical distinction between psoriasis vulgaris and pustular psoriasis is supported by the observation that only the former shows association with

HLA. However, the associations may be used also to tie together related diseases, such as ankylosing spondylitis, Reiter's disease, some other postinfectious arthropathies, acute anterior uveitis, and balanitis, which all show association with HLA-B27. This points to a common pathogenic pathway in these disorders, although they affect different organs. In analogy, the associations between HLA-Dw3 and Addison's disease, Graves' disease, and insulin-independent diabetes, confirm the concept that these three disorders are related: they belong to the so-called organ-specific autoimmune diseases. However, it is worth noting that Hashimoto's thyroiditis and pernicious anemia are apparently not associated with HLA-Dw3, although they too have been considered members of this group, which again illustrates the usefulness of HLA studies in disease classification.

V. Inheritance of Disease Susceptibility and Resistance

Apart from C2 deficiency and 21-hydroxylase deficiency, none of the diseases listed in Table II have a simple mode of inheritance. In some cases, e.g., multiple sclerosis, prior investigations have shown that there is a higher frequency of the disease among the relatives of the patients than in the general population, but it is worth noting that family aggregation of a disease is no proof of a genetic background: such aggregation may also be explained by the possibility that relatives share environmental factors more often than do unrelated individuals. When twin studies have been carried out, they have usually shown that there is not complete concordance in monozygotic twins, which reflects incomplete penetrance and indicates that environmental factors also play a role in the development of the disease. Indeed, this lack of complete penetrance and a varying age at onset has been one of the major obstacles to a clarification of the inheritance of disease susceptibility. Now the HLA associations finally prove that there is a genetic susceptibility to all disorders listed in Table II. The HLA antigens are genetic markers associated with disease susceptibility and provide a new tool in such genetic studies. Nevertheless, it should be mentioned that these studies are somewhat hampered by the fact that we still do not know which HLA factors are truly responsible for the disease liability. This may not be the antigens listed in Table II, but could be still unknown HLA factors associated with those now known to be related to the diseases. As discussed in by Rubinstein in this volume, such nonrandom association or linkage disequilibrium between HLA factors is a well known phenomenon in the general population. Still, even with this reservation in mind, the presently known disease associations have already yielded important information about the inheritance of disease susceptibility. The clearest example is ankylosing spondylitis, where HLA-B27—or another HLA factor very closely associated with B27—confers a strong susceptibility to the disease. Moreover, this susceptibility must be inherited mainly as a dominant trait, as the risk of ankylosing spondylitis is approximately the same for *B27* heterozygotes as for *B27* homozygotes. It is of interest to note that studies of apparently healthy B27-positive individuals have revealed a striking prevalence (about 20%) of nonsymptomatic sacroileitis both in males and in females, although classical ankylosing spondylitis occurs about five times more frequently in males than in females.

The inheritance of diabetes has been called the nightmare of the geneticist. One major reason why this problem has been so difficult to solve is that distinction often has not been made between juvenile and maturity-onset diabetes. It is now clear that these two groups must be treated separately. Another difficulty has been the lack of genetic factors associated with the disease. Not fewer than three such factors are now available for insulin-dependent diabetes. One of these factors, HLA-Dw2, provides an extraordinary protection against this disease, while two other HLA antigens, HLA-Dw3 and Dw4, confer quite strong susceptibility. Thus, it seems that three different HLA factors may be responsible for at least part of the genetic susceptibility to insulin-dependent diabetes. However, it is also possible that this susceptibility is due to the action of just one HLA factor, which must then be particularly frequent in haplotypes carrying Dw3 or Dw4 and extremely rare in Dw2 haplotypes. Studies are in progress to clarify which of these possibilities is correct.

HLA studies in families with more than one affected relative provide important information in addition to that inherent in the association data. For example, it has recently been shown that there is an excess of HLA identity among sib pairs both of whom suffer from hemochromatosis, and this indicates that hemachromatosis is inherited as a recessive trait.

For most of the other diseases listed in Table II, the information inherent in the HLA associations has not yet been fully explored in terms of classifying the mode of inheritance.

VI. Mechanisms that Can Explain the Associations

The increasing knowledge about the biological functions of the HLA system adds another aspect to the HLA and disease associations, as it may point to specific pathogenic mechanisms in these disorders, the causes of which are for the most part unknown at the present time. Most of our knowledge about the biological functions of major histocompatibility complexes (MHCs), such as the HLA system, derives from animal studies, but as there is a striking homology between MHCs in all species, there is little doubt that the findings in these studies hold for the HLA system too. Here, we will mention only the most important points. The MHC controls a variety of specific immune responses, in particular the development of cell-mediated immunity and the production of IgG antibodies. In the species studied, the immune response (*Ir*) genes responsible for this action have been located very close to the homolog of the *HLA-D/DR* genes in man. The HLA-ABC antigens and their homologs in animals play a role as part of the targets in the immune lysis of virus-infected and hapten-conjugated cells. Finally, the MHC controls some of the complement components, which are important for the elimination of infectious microorganisms.

When speculating about the mechanisms that can explain the disease associations, it seems reasonable to assume that relationships primarily involving HLA-D and DR antigens are due to the action of specific *Ir* genes, while those involving HLA-ABC antigens may reflect a specific effector phase of cell-mediated immunity. The first of these assumptions is supported by the fact that most of the HLA-D-associated diseases listed in Table II are characterized by elements of autoimmunity. Thus, organ-specific autoimmune antibodies directed against the affected organ can often be demonstrated in the Sicca syndrome, insulin-dependent diabetes, and Addison's disease, among others. Indeed, antiadrenal autoantibodies have been shown to occur significantly more frequently in HLA-Dw3-positive patients with Addison's disease than in Dw3-negative patients. In celiac disease and dermatitis herpetiformis hypersensitivity to gluten seems to play a major role in the pathogenesis, and the association with HLA-Dw3 could reflect the effect of an Ir determinant with specificity for some component in gluten.

Molecular mimicry is another mechanism that has been suggested as an explanation for the relationship between HLA and disease. According to this hypothesis, it is assumed that similarity between a microbial antigen and an HLA antigen may render individuals carrying this HLA antigen more susceptible to infection than others. This mechanism has been suggested as an explanation for the association between HLA-B27 and ankylosing spondylitis. However, although this is an attractive theory, there is not much evidence to support it at the present time.

Apart from the association between Dw2 deficiency and C2-deficiency, which can lead to lupus-like syndromes, it does not seem likely that complement abnormalities are responsible for other presently known diseases associations.

The strong association between HLA-A3 and idiopathic hemochromatosis indicates that immune mechanisms may not always be the basis for associations between HLA and disease. Idiopathic hemochromatosis is characterized by an abnormally high uptake of iron from the gut, and there is no evidence of aberrant immunity. The relationship to HLA suggests that the HLA system plays a role also in some biological phenomena not involving the immune system.

VII. Diagnostic and Prognostic Value

As mentioned in the Introduction, HLA typing has already found a place as a diagnostic aid for a few of the HLA-associated diseases. Thus, investigation for HLA-B27 has been of clinical value in unclear early cases of suspected ankylosing spondylitis, sacroileitis, or Reiter's disease. For example, in ankylosing spondylitis, HLA-B27 typing may be considered to be a diagnostic test with about 9% false positives and about 90% negatives. It is worth noting that the value of HLA typing depends on the a priori probability of the disease based on other clinical findings. With an a priori probability of ankylosing spondylitis of about 50%, the posteriori probabilities are 90% or 10% if the patient is HLA-B27 positive or negative, respectively.

It is also possible that HLA typing may have prognostic value. For example, multiple sclerosis seems to run a more severe course in Dw2-positive as compared to Dw2-negative patients, and the same may be true of rheumatoid arthritis in Dw4-positive patients. Moreover, there is evidence that thryotoxicosis treated with antithyroid drugs is more likely to relapse in Dw3-positive than in Dw3-negative patients. However, more studies are needed to establish these relationships.

Finally, it may be added that some of the relationships between HLA and diseases may also prove to be valuable in genetic counseling (e.g., in juvenile diabetes), but it is still too early to evaluate this possibility.

Acknowledgments

This work was supported by the Danish Medical Research Council and the Medical Research council of EEC. Our thanks are due to Mrs. Elly Andersen for expert secretarial assistance.

Key References

Dausset, J., and Svejgaard, A., eds. (1977). "HLA Disease." Munksgaard, Copenhagen.
Ryder, L. P., Andersen, E., and Svejgaard, A. (1979). "HLA and Disease Registry, Third Report." Munksgaard, Copenhagen.
Svejgaard, A., Hauge, M., Jersild, C., Platz, P., Ryder, L. P., Staub Nielsen, L., and Thomsen, M. (1979). "The HLA System—An Introductory Survey" (second revised edition) (*Monogr. Human Genet.* 7). Karger, Basel.
Svejgaard, A., Platz, P., and Ryder, L. P. (1977). Associations between HLA and some non-rheumatic diseases and possible explanations. *In* "Immunogenetics and Rheumatic Disease—" (D. A. Brewerton, ed.), *Clinics in Rheumatic Disease* **3,** 239–253.

Other Markers in the HLA Linkage Group[1]

PABLO RUBINSTEIN

The Lindsley F. Kimball Research Institute of The New York Blood Center, Inc.,
New York, New York

I. Introduction	183
II. Genetic Considerations	185
III. Other Markers in the HLA Linkage Group	186
IV. Complement Components	187
A. Factor B of Properdin or Bf	187
B. The Second Component of Complement (C2)	188
C. The Fourth Component of Complement (C4)	189
D. Other Components of Complement	191
V. Intracellular Enzymes	191
A. Phosphoglucomutase-3	192
B. Glyoxalase-1	192
C. 21-Hydroxylase	193
VI. Concluding Remarks	193
Selected References	194

I. Introduction

In 1967, at the Third International Workshop on Histocompatibility Testing, it was reported that the distribution of HLA antigens (in particular the antigen then called 4c) among patients with Hodgkin's disease differed significantly from that among normal controls. This ob-

---

[1]This work was supported in part by grants HL 09011 and AM 19631 from the National Institutes of Health.

servation triggered an enormous interest among researchers in the HLA field that focused on the proposition that particular HLA types may be important in determining the likelihood that their carriers may develop (or resist the development of) specific diseases. The results of this interest are of such magnitude that it has been necessary to organize a computer-based International Registry on HLA and disease.

Most of the work in this area has been directed at establishing statistical associations between an antigen and a disease, but obviously considerable interest exists in the exploration of the mechanisms leading to the abnormal distribution of HLA antigens in patients with such diseases. One of the most generally blamed possible mechanisms involves "immune response" genes in the pathogenesis of these conditions. This hypothesis involves, among others, the assumptions that immune response genes exist in man and that they are closely linked to the HLA region. Most important, it is implicit in the hypothesis that the alleles of the immune response genes associate preferentially with specific HLA region alleles, i.e., that the two regions maintain significant linkage disequilibrium. (Linkage in genetic terms refers to the physical proximity of two genes located in the same chromosome, which results in nonindependent segregation of the traits inherited through them. Alleles at linked loci are expected to arrive at equilibrium with one another, that is, to form combinations called haplotypes with a frequency equal to the product of their respective gene frequencies. When this equilibrium is not obtained and specific alleles at the two loci occur together with a significantly increased or decreased frequency, these alleles are said to be in "linkage disequilibrium.")

HLA may be involved directly in the determination of disease susceptibility, rather than through the effects of linked genes. If, for example, one of the main antigens on a pathogenic microorganism is immunochemically similar to a given HLA antigen, carriers of that antigen may have increased risk of infection and/or of severity of disease: this is called molecular mimicry. A more complex mechanism of direct antigenic involvement may be mediated by the restriction phenomenon: the efficiency of target-cell destruction by specific killer lymphocytes is much higher when killer and target share the major histocompatibility antigens. The phenomenon is particularly striking when the targets are virus-infected cells: HLA antigens, therefore, must play an important role in the defense against cellular parasites.

Beyond the effects of the HLA genes themselves and of the immune response genes assumed to map in the HLA region, the genetic background for the association between HLA and diseases must be provided by other genes located close to this region. This chapter will explore the "other" genes currently known to be linked to the HLA and will examine the methodology used in the genetic analysis of linkage.

II. Genetic Considerations

The number of structural genes believed to exist in man is of the order of 50,000. This exceeds by three orders of magnitude the number of human chromosomes and it is clear that many genes must be carried by each chromosome. The spots at which genes occur (loci) are arranged in longitudinal sequences so that some loci are adjacent to one another while others in the same chromosome may be much farther apart. The proximity of two genetic loci, therefore, need not have special significance per se, but it may provide information of both practical and theoretical interest, as we shall see.

The classical method for the investigation of linkage between two genetic loci is the analysis of segregation patterns in informative families. If the loci are not in fact linked, half of the children of a doubly heterozygous parent married to a homozygous individual will inherit both genes together; if they are linked, significantly more than 50% of the children will receive them both. If they are very closely linked, they will segregate together in essentially 100% of the time. The analysis of segregation data consists of comparing the probability with which the observed pattern would result if the genes are linked with the probability with which it would occur if they are not. The comparison is usually made with the lod-score method (lod = logarithm of the odds), which is essentially the logarithm of the ratio between the two probabilities. Different ratios may be expected depending on the genetic distance between the two loci, which can be estimated from the percentage of times that they are separated by crossing-over. For this reason it is useful to calculate the lod scores for a series of possible values of the recombination fraction (θ). Logarithms are used so that the values from individual families may be conveniently added. Lod scores of 3 are considered sufficient to establish linkage, as the likelihood of linkage is then 1000-fold greater than that of independent segregation. Similarly, a score of -2 establishes absence of linkage.

The study of segregation in families is limited to those traits that exhibit genetic variants, i.e., characters or structures that may occur in different forms in individuals of the same species. The species is said to be polymorphic with regard to the trait in question. The classical examples of genetic variants are the ABO blood group antigens in humans. This trait, the ABO blood group, is determined by a single locus with three main alleles, A, B, and O, the phenotypic effects of which are the ABO antigens. Chemical studies have shown that the O blood group results from the absence of a terminal sugar moiety in the glycoprotein that expresses ABO specificities: O could thus be thought of as a "null" allele and the O blood group as a deficiency state. Deficiency states, therefore, may be used as genetic variants in the study of segregation and linkage, provided of course, that they are not lethal. The study of inherited deficiencies may be complicated because more than one genetic mechanism may result in the deficiency of the same character. The Rh-null phenotype, for example—that is, the inherited absence of all Rh antigens—has been seen to be caused by a gene allelic to the "normal" *Rh* genes and also by an independently segregating one. Inherited deficiencies, therefore, are not necessarily variants of the same genetic locus even if they result in identical phenotypes. Awareness of this fact is important when studying the linkage relationships of a gene through inherited deficiencies of its products in different families.

III. Other Markers in the HLA Linkage Group

The HLA system itself is currently defined by the products of at least four loci, A, B, C, and D. The first three determine serologically detectable antigens present in essentially all nucleated cells while *HLA-D*-determined antigens are expressed in just a few types of cells: B lymphocytes, sperm, and some epidermal cells are the best studied ones. The serological expression of *HLA-D*, called HLA-DR (for D-related) antigens, appears to be very closely associated if not identical with the HLA-D specificities defined with the classical mixed lymphocyte culture (MLC) procedures described elsewhere in this volume. Each of these four loci possesses a large number of alleles, and consequently each chromosome 6 has a very high probability of displaying a different combination of alleles at the four loci from that carried by its paired homolog. Thus almost every family permits us to identify all four HLA regions (haplotypes) present in the parents and to follow their segregation. If a genetic variant of any trait is segregating in a given pedigree, therefore, one can very nearly always study whether it segregates together with HLA. Other genetic markers are not so polymorphic, and for this reason alone the linkage of genes close to HLA may be uncovered much more easily than is the case for other linkage groups.

Linkage between HLA and several other loci has in fact been demonstrated. These other genes appear to determine either components of the complement system or intracellular enzymes. As we shall see, four or five loci that control the C3-activating components and three genes that control enzymes without apparent relationship to each other or to the major histocompatibility system have been found to map in or close to this genetic region. We shall now describe the most salient aspects of these traits and will attempt to put their linkage to HLA in a biological perspective.

IV. Complement Components

Three complement components, Bf, C2, and C4, are inherited through genes in the HLA linkage group. Bf was mapped because it presents electrophoretic variants; C2 and C4 exhibit both electrophoretic polymorphism and inherited deficiency states. In the case of C4, most exciting evidences for linkage to HLA were contributed by the study of the blood group antigens Chido (Ch a) and Rodgers (Rg a).

A. Factor B of Properdin or Bf

This complement component, formerly called GBG (for glycine-rich βglobulin), was the first to be mapped in the HLA region. Bf is identical to C3PA (C3 proactivator), a component of the properdin pathway of the activation of C3 and of its amplification loop. The variants of Bf are discernible by serum electrophoresis in agarose followed by immunofixation with specific anti-Bf antibody (usually made in goats). Four alleles have been identified: *Bf S*, *F*, *Fl*, and *Sl*, in order of frequency in Caucasion populations. The location of *Bf* is very close to that of *HLA*: in the original investigation, no instance of recombination between these loci was found. The exact position of *Bf* relative to the *HLA* loci is not completely clear. The study of a number of families with intra-HLA recombinations appears to favor the order: *HLA-A*,

HLA-C, *HLA-B*, *Bf*, *HLA-D*, since crossing-overs that separate *HLA-B* from *HLA-D* leave *Bf* with *HLA-B* in some families and with *HLA-D* in others. Other reports do not fit this scheme and more information is clearly required on this point. There is evidence of linkage disequilibrium between alleles at the *Bf* and *HLA* loci: the strongest one links *Bf F1* with *HLA-B18*, while *Bf F* is associated with *HLA-B12*. *Bf F1* may also be in linkage disequilibrium with juvenile diabetes, although this information has been obtained in France, where *HLA-B18* is associated with this disease, and the disequilibrium may therefore be secondary to that between *HLA-B18* and juvenile diabetes.

B. THE SECOND COMPONENT OF COMPLEMENT (C2)

Mapping of the locus (or loci) that determine or control the synthesis of C2 has been possible using either the electrophoretic variants or the deficiency as genetic markers.

1. C2 Deficiency

Deficiency of C2 is inherited as a recessive character. The gene responsible, $C2°$, segregates in close linkage to *HLA* and was the second of the complement components to be mapped in this region. Ascertainment of the presence of $C2°$ is based in the complete absence of C2 in the serum by both functional and immunochemical tests while the rest of the complement components are essentially undisturbed. This consideration is important because several pathological conditions, especially some autoimmune processes, may lead to *in vivo* activation of the complement cascade and to consumption of several components. This constitutes an "acquired deficiency" and may be troublesome because the inherited deficiency state itself is often associated with a lupus-like syndrome. When $C2°$ is present in single dose, ($C2°$-heterozygous condition) the levels of C2 in the serum are reduced. Because the normal levels of C2 have a very wide range, however, definition of the heterozygous state is far more reliable when it is made in the family of a $C2°$-homozygote. Quantitation of serum C2 is carried out by functional and/or immunochemical tests, which should both be used in the study of the possibly C2-deficient patient. It appears that immunochemical quantitation has lower variances than do functional procedures and may be more reliable for the detection of $C2°$ heterozygotes.

The families of about 20 C2-deficient individuals have been typed for HLA. In addition to the demonstration of close linkage, these studies disclosed the existence of linkage disequilibrium between $C2°$ and the HLA haplotype *A25, B18, Dw2*. This disequilibrium is remarkable on several accounts; the HLA haplotype in question is not in such strong linkage disequilibrium in the absence of $C2°$, and furthermore the two loci have been observed to be separated by crossing-over with a frequency of 2–4%. It has been suggested for these reasons that the $C2°$ mutation may have occurred in a single *HLA-A25, B18, Dw2* haplotype from which it spread to the different families in which it has been encountered. The fact that in all cases the "carrier" haplotype also determines Bf S may, too, be due to its common origin.

2. C2 Polymorphism

Two common electrophoretic variants of C2 have been encountered, and a number of rarer ones, the genes for all of which segregate as alleles at a single locus. No recombinations between this locus and *HLA* have been found which contrasts with the observations described above for C2 deficiency. This puzzling phenomenon suggests that the locus that controls the synthesis (and, thus, the electrophoretic mobility) of C2 is different from that at which the $C2°$ mutant occurs. It is, however, possible that $C2°$ represents a structural gene mutant and that the difference in the recombination frequency reflects some sort of chromosomal instability caused by the mutation itself.

The technique for C2 typing is not simple: the first step is electrofocusing on acrylamide gels after which a gellified medium containing optimally sensitized sheep erythrocytes and C2-deficient serum is layered on top. The position of the separated C2 is revealed by localized areas of hemolysis in the overlay.

C. The Fourth Component of Complement (C4)

Three types of genetic markers have been used in the family studies that disclosed the location of this component in the HLA region: the gene that causes C4 deficiency $C4°$, the electrophoretic variants of C4, and the blood group antigens Chido (Ch a) and Rodgers (Rg a) now known to be parts of C4.

Ch a and Rg a

Chido was described in 1967 as a "nebulous" antibody that produced difficulties in cross-matching blood for transfusion. The nebulous nature of the antibody is due to the very marked differences in the agglutinability of the red cells of different Ch a-positive individuals and to the rather weak agglutination that is obtained even when the titer of the antiserum is very high. The serum of Ch a-positive individuals, however, inhibits the agglutination reaction; that is, the antigen is present in serum, which permits us to bypass the serological problem by choosing strongly reacting red cells as targets for the test. Linkage tests were also hindered by the large differences in the frequency of the two alleles, Ch (a+) and Ch (a−), and by the dominance of Ch (a+), which makes the Ch (a+) homozygous individuals phenotypically identical to the heterozygous. Only about 2% of Caucasians are Ch (a−). In spite of these difficulties it has been possible to demonstrate very close linkage between *Chido* and *HLA*. The *Chido* locus in fact appears to be "inside" *HLA* since intra-HLA crossovers place it sometimes with the *D* locus and others with *HLA-B*. Strong linkage disequilibrium exists between the Ch (a−) allele and the HLA-B alleles *B12*, *Bw35*, and *B5*.

The Rodgers blood group is also inherited *en bloc* with the HLA system. Again this is a serum antigen, and just as for Chido, Rodgers typing is much more reliable when performed by the serum inhibition technique. Both Ch (a) and Rg (a) may be acquired by Ch (a−) and Rg (a−) red cells upon transfusion to positive individuals. *Rg (a−)* is also in linkage disequilibrium with *HLA-B*, specifically with *HLA-B8*. Although both Chido and Rodgers are linked to HLA and in spite of their very similar phenotypic appearance, the two are not allelic to each other, and the significance of this fact became clear when it was found that the Chido and Rodgers substances in serum are parts of C4. This finding culminates a most interesting series of observations, which began in 1975 with the discovery of linkage between HLA and the gene that causes the inherited deficiency of C4 ($C4°$). One year later, electrophoretic variants of C4 were described using anti-C4 antibodies to precipitate the electrophoretically separated C4 bands (immunofixation). The variants were difficult to analyze, as the resulting phenotypes were not too distinct. Two main alleles at a single locus closely linked to HLA were inferred, however, which appeared to segregate in the expected manner. The original report has received confirmation from other workers while still others could not reproduce the technique with similar results. The cause of the discrepancies may have been related to the spontaneous activation of C4 that occurs in serum. When EDTA-plasma was used instead of serum, a different picture emerged. The electrophoretic patterns became much more clearly defined and suggested the presence of genes at closely linked loci, rather than of allelic genes. The conclusion that C4 consists of the products of two separate genes was made all the more exciting by the fact that the absence of the electrophoretically fast component occurs always (and only) in individuals that are Rg (a−). Similarly, absence of the slow component is invariably accompanied by the Ch (a−) status. Moreover, individuals who are C4 deficient are invariably Ch (a−) *and* Rg (a−). All these associations would be extremely unlikely unless Chido and Rodgers are indeed molecular components of C4. Thus, additionally, Chido and Rodgers became the first blood groups the biological roles of which are directly elucidated.

D. Other Components of Complement

The linkage of Bf, C2, and C4 to HLA triggered a search for linkage of other complement components. The results obtained by several different groups of investigators, however, established the independent segregation of HLA from the electrophoretic variants of C3, C6, and C7 and from the deficiencies of C1r, C1s-inhibitor, and C8. In the case of C8, an early claim of linkage to HLA has not been upheld. Thus, it appears that only the three components that are physiologically involved in the activation of C3 are linked to HLA. Unraveling of the physiological significance of the genetic association of the major histocompatibility system with the C3 proactivators should be of interest for our understanding not only of the regulation of complement activation, but also of the evolutionary influence of linkage.

V. Intracellular Enzymes

Three enzymes have been mapped close to the HLA region: phosphoglucomutase-3 (PGM-3), glyoxalase-1 (GLO), and 21-hydroxylase. The first two could be studied because of the existence of electrophoretic allotypes, and the third because of the availability of families with inherited deficiencies.

A. Phosphoglucomutase-3

Three different enzymes may be detected in cells that have phosphoglucomutase activity. PGM-1 and PGM-2 are expressed very well in red cells, but PGM-3 can be demonstrated only in nucleated cells, mainly in placental tissue and lymphocytes. Lysates from such cells are subjected to electrophoresis in agarose gels after which the enzymic activity is elicited by overlaying the gels with appropriate reagents. The mobility of the colored bands is then estimated by reference to standards. The locus responsible for these variants has been mapped in the HLA region, but at a relatively large distance: the recombination fraction is about 17% in males. As with other autosomal linkages, the recombination in females is more frequent; therefore, the linkage to HLA is not demonstrable in families in which the mother is the PGM-3-heterozygous parent. The position of *PGM-3* in the chromosome has been determined more precisely: this locus is between *HLA-D* and the centromere.

B. Glyoxalase-1

Glyoxalase-1 also exhibits electrophoretic variants: a fast (F) and a slow (S) allele have been described in red cell lysates. Recently a "null" allele has been identified, although no homozygous deficient individuals have yet been found. The technique is comparatively simple, and because the enzyme is detectable in stored erythrocytes, studies of this polymorphism are greatly facilitated. The position of *GLO* relative to *HLA* has been established by families with intra-HLA recombinations: it maps between *HLA-D* and *PGM-3*. The actual distance between *HLA* and *GLO* is somewhat uncertain. The original estimate was about 10% for the recombination fraction; others are as low as 3%. in our own material the frequency of recombination is 5% in males and 9% in females.

No linkage disequilibrium has been found between *HLA* and *GLO* alleles, which may not be surprising in view of the rather large distance between these loci. On the other hand, murine *GLO* is linked to *H-2*, the homolog of HLA in mice. Because of the persistence of this linkage in evolution, one might expect some type of functional association to exist between these loci. Again, the exploration of this association should provide insights into some of the most basic questions regarding the evolutionary influence of linkage.

Be this as it may, *GLO* has proved a very useful marker in the study of intra-HLA recombinations because of its position closely "outside" *HLA-D*. In informative cases *GLO* may prove an otherwise doubtful crossing-over.

C. 21-Hydroxylase

The inherited deficiency of this enzyme is the most frequent cause of congenital adrenal hyperplasia through its effect on the synthesis of cortisol. This recessive condition is the first inborn error of metabolism to be found in linkage with HLA: in a number of families with two affected children the probands shared invariably *both* HLA haplotypes. The lod score in this material was significantly over 3 at a recombination fraction of 0; in other words, linkage is very close. Intra-HLA recombinants place this locus in a position adjacent to HLA-B, that is, within HLA. The families reported so far provide additional information: no instance of consanguinity was reported, which indicates that the frequency of the deficiency gene is not very low. This is confirmed by the fact that the two haplotypes of the affected children were different from each other in all cases. Additionally, there is no evidence of linkage disequilibrium with particular HLA alleles. Besides its obvious interest in associating HLA to the genes that control the synthesis of adrenal hormones, this linkage may have an importnat practical application. By HLA-typing the amniotic cells of fetuses in families where a case has already been observed, it may be possible to identify antenatally individuals homozygous for the deficiency gene.

VI. Concluding Remarks

The existence of linkage between apparently unrelated traits carries with it the possibility that reasons may be uncovered that answer the teleological question: Why are these traits linked?

One such reason is already available: Chido and Rodgers are linked to the major histocompatibility system because they are really the genes that control the synthesis of the two components of C4. The more general aspect of this question is why are the C3 proactivators linked to HLA. A beginning of an answer may be provided by the study of the role of C3 on at lease some H-2-controlled T–B cell interactions in mice.

Much less clear are the reasons behind the linkage of the genes for the enzymes reviewed above. The extreme tightness of the linkage between HLA and 21-hydroxylase may imply that reasons do exist. Although androgen metabolism in mice is partly controlled by genes in the *H-2* region, the biological significance of this is not at all understood. In the case of GLO we have proof that the linkage relationships transcend species barriers, but we are equally in the dark as to the functional implications of this close genetic association. Even less is known about PGM-3: the linkage of the locus for PGM-3 to HLA may be entirely coincidental, as suggested by the relatively large distance between them.

We do not know, therefore, how, or even whether, these "other" genes in the HLA region are associated with the susceptibility to specific diseases, except in the case of C2 deficiency and the *HLA-A25,B18, Dw2* haplotype and C4 deficiency and Chido–Rodgers negativity. We can expect, however, that the exploration of their functional association with the immunological aspects of HLA may provide insight into the mechanisms behind some of the HLA-disease associations. In the last analysis, it is the understanding of the biology of linkage that will provide answers to the question of how and why susceptibility to a disease is determined by the HLA phenotype.

Selected References

Bach, F. H., and van Rood, J. J (1976). The major histocompatibility complex—Genetics and biology (in three parts). *N. Engl. J. Med.* **295**, 806–813, 872–878, 927–936.

Crow, J. F., and Kimura, M. (1970). "An Introduction to Population Genetics Theory." Harper, New York.

Giblett, E. R. (1969). "Genetic Markers in Human Blood." Blackwell, Oxford.

Jersild, C., Rubinstein, P., and Day, N. K. (1976). The HLA system and inherited deficiencies of the complement system. *Transplant. Rev.* **32**, 43–71.

Müller-Eberhard, H. J. (1975). Complement. *Annu. Rev. Biochem.* **44**, 697–724.

Race, R. R., and Sanger, R. (1975). "Blood Groups in Man," 6th ed. Blackwell, Oxford.

Index

A
Antigens, B cell differentiation and, 11

B
B cell, differentiation antigens, 11

C
Cell surface, of lymphocyte populations, markers on, 3–4
Chronic lymphatic leukemia, lymphocytes, expression of C receptors on, 41–42
Complement, components, HLA linkage group and, 187–191
Complement receptors, 33–37
    expression of on lymphocytes
        from CLL patients, 41–42
        from macroglobulinema patients, 42
        from normal blood, 40–41
        interpretation and significance, 42–45
        of lymphocyte membrane, in tonsils, spleen and thoracic duct, 42
    of lymphocyte subpopulations, 13–14
    methods of detection
        fluorescence assays, 38–39
        rosette assays, 37–38
        specificity controls, 39

Cytotoxicity, natural, specificity of, 79–82

D
Disease, HLA and, 173–174
    diagnostic and prognostic value, 180–181
    disease heterogeneity, 176–177
    inheritance of disease susceptibility and resistance, 177–178
    mechanisms explaining associations, 179–180
    methods, 174–175
    relationships between HLA and diseases, 175–176

G
Glyoxalase-1, HLA linkage group and, 192–193
Graft survival, HLA and, 161–164
    discussion, 169–171
    methodology, 164–166
    results, 166–169

H
HLA
    disease and, 173–174

diagnostic and prognostic value, 180–181
disease heterogeneity, 176–177
graft survival and, 161–164
discussion, 169–171
methodology, 164–166
results, 166–169
inheritance of disease susceptibility and resistance, 177–178
mechanisms explaining associations, 179–180
methods, 174–175
relationships between HLA and diseases, 175–176
HLA-D region encoded antigens, definition by T lymphocyte reactivities
general discussion, 141–142
mixed leukocyte culture with homozygous typing cells, 127–132
primed LD-typing, 132–141
HLA-DR, serology of, 113–114
discussion, 120–121
results, 118–120
technical considerations, 114–118
HLA linkage group
complement components in
factor B of properdin or Bf, 187–188
fourth component, 189–191
other components, 191
second component, 188–189
genetic considerations, 185–186
intracellular enzymes and, 191–192
glyoxalase-1, 192–193
21-hydroxylase, 193
phosphoglucomutase-3, 192
other markers in, 186–187
HLApA, -B and -C, serology of, 99–100
conclusions, 109–111
experimental methods and findings, 100–103
21-Hydroxylase, HLA linkage group and, 193

I

Immune system, regulation by lymphocyte sets
analysis in the mouse, 91–95
conclusions, 95–97
general considerations, 89–91
Immunoglobulin(s), lymphocyte membrane
changes in, 7
classes of, 6–7
methods and technical problems, 8–9
Immunoglobulin A, Fc receptor of, 16
Immunoglobulin D, Fc receptor of, 17
Immunoglobulin E, Fc receptor of, 16–17
Immunoglobulin G, Fc receptor of, 14–15
Immunoglobulin M, Fc receptor of, 16

K

Killer cells, factors affecting levels of activity, 82–83

L

Lectins, clinical usefulness of, 65–67
abnormalities at level of macrophages, 69
imbalances in regulatory T cells, 69–72
influence of soluble serum factors, 67–69
Leukocyte(s), mixed culture
homozygous typing cells, 127–128
methods, 127
results, 128–132
Lymphocyte(s), lectin-induced activation, procedures for determining in vitro, 62–65
Lymphocyte membrane, complement receptors
expression of, 40–42
interpretation and significance, 42–45
methods of detection, 37–39
Lymphocyte populations, 4–5
Lymphocyte sets, immune system regulation by
analysis in the mouse, 91–95
conclusions, 95–97
general considerations, 89–91
Lymphocyte subpopulations
background, 2–3
complement receptors, 13–14
cytoplasmic immunoglobulins, 5–6
distinction from monocytes, 28–29

enzymatic markers
  acid phosphatase, 18
  α-napthyl acetate esterase, 17–18
  terminal deoxynucleotidyl transferase, 18
Epstein–Barr virus receptor, 12–13
erythrocyte receptors
  for *Macaca speciosa* monkey RBC
  for mouse receptors
  for rhesus monkey
  for SRBC
Ia system
  background, 9–10
  cellular distinction, 11–12
  methods of detection, 10
markers on cell surface, 3
membrane immunoglobulins
  changes in, 7–8
  classes, 6–7
  methods and technical problems, 8–9
receptors for Fc region of immunoglobulin
  the IgA Fc receptor, 16
  the IgD Fc receptor, 17
  the IgE Fc receptor, 16–17
  the IgG Fc receptor, 14–15
  the IgM Fc receptor, 16
receptors for peanut agglutinin, 18–19
surface antigens of, defined by monoclonal antibodies
  background, 21–23
  monoclonal antibodies, 23–26
  clinical application of, 25–26
Lympholysis, cell-mediated, 143–144
  future prospects, 158–159
  genetic control of, 148–151
  preliminary information from typing, 157–158
  specificity, 147–148
  technique, 146–147
  terminology, 145–146
  typing, 151–157

M

Macroglobulinemia, lymphocytes, expression of C receptors on, 42

Macrophages, abnormalities, lectins and, 69
Mitogenesis, lectin-induced, fundamentals of, 57–62
Monocytes,
  distinction from lymphocytes, 16–17
  relationship with Tγ cells, 26–28

N

Natural killer cells characteristics and relationship to K cells, 77–79
  factors affecting levels of activity, 82–83
  methods, 74–77
  possible clinical significance of, 84–86

P

Phosphoglucomutase-3, HLA linkage group and, 192
Primed LD-typing
  discussion, 140–141
  methods, 132–134
  pool-PLT, 138–140
  results, 134–138

S

Serology of HLA-DR, 113–114
  discussion, 120–121
  results, 118–120
  technical considerations, 114–118
Serology of HLApA, -B and -C, 99–100
  conclusions, 109–111
  experimental methods and findings, 100–103
Serum factors, usefulness of lectins and, 67–69
Spleen, CRL in, 42

T

T cells
  definition of HLA-D region encoded antigens
    general discussion, 141–142
    mixed leukocyte culture with homozygous typing cells, 127–132

primed LD-typing, 132–141
regulatory, lectins and, 69–72
$T_{·G}$ cells
  enumeration and isolation of, 48–49
  functional analysis of, 50–52
  morphology of, 49
  subpopulation
    clinical relevance of, 52–53
  tissue distribution of, 50
Tγ cells, relationship with monocytes, 26–28, *see also* $T_{·G}$ cells
$T_{·M}$ cells
  functional analysis of, 50–52
  isolation and enumeration, 48–49
  morphology of, 49
  subpopulation
    clinical relevance of, 52–53
  tissue distribution of, 50
Third-cell population (unclassified lymphoid cells), 29–30
Thoracic duct, CRL in, 42
T lymphocytes, *see* T cells
Tonsils, CRL in, 42
Typing, cell-mediated lympholysis and, 151–155
  analysis of specificity of cytotoxic lymphocytes, 155–156
  definition of positive and negative results, 154–155
  procurement of cytotoxic typing lymphocytes, 153–154
  selection of cells identical for new target specificities, 156–157
  standardized target cell panels, 154